'At turns hilarious, horrifying and always painfully honest, [this] is a memoir about how one woman 'gained a baby and lost her shit.' This is the side of motherhood and what it can do to your mental health and your labia that isn't covered in NCT classes.'
SARRA MANNING, *Red Magazine*

'A spit-out-your-tea funny chronicle of becoming a mum for the first time, from the awkwardness of making friends on maternity leave to the politics of post-baby sex. A great read.'
Marie Claire

'An honest take on the way we approach and define motherhood. It made me laugh and Grace is a refreshing voice on the subject.'
LORRAINE CANDY, *Sunday Times Style*

'Hilarious in parts, poignant in others, reading Grace's musings on motherhood felt like stumbling across the diary of a witty classmate. I wanted to hug her, thank her for reassuring me that I'm not alone in questioning my self-identity as a mother and then I wanted to invite her to the pub so we could chat about pregnancy wind and post-birth coital relations. Five stars plus a little bit of laughter-wee.'
SARAH TURNER, author of *The Unmumsy Mum*

'I howled with laughter   *re*

'Honestly brilliant'   E   *e*

'This is the best book my daughter ever wrote about her vagina.'
CHRISTOPHER TIMOTHY

'Grace takes a deeper, more raw look at what being a mother means for a modern woman. Like Bryony Gordon did for the twenty-somethings in the *Wrong Knickers*, Grace has now shone a similarly funny and candid light on motherhood. She has managed to express exactly how I felt as a new mum, but in the way you'd like your funniest motherhood anecdote to be told.'

HELEN WHITAKER, author of *The School Run*

'A friend of mine just had her first baby. I didn't send her champagne or flowers or breast pads. I sent her Grace's book. I'm now that baby's godmother. It's that good.' GEORGIA TENNANT

'Low on data but high on empathy, this is the memoir on the overwhelming identity crisis that becoming a mother can be.'

The Pool

'This book absolutely blew me away.' RUTH CRILLY

'Grace writes with wicked wit and real emotional resonance too – even though I'm not a mother I related deeply to her exploration of what it's like to navigate the world as a woman, and the expectations that are placed upon us all.'

DAISY BUCHANAN, author of *How To Be A Grown Up*

'Brilliant!' CLEMMIE TELFORD

'Such a good read, even for us dads. There's talk of vaginas, babies, IKEA chairs and, er, more vaginas.' JAMIE DAY

ABOUT THE AUTHOR

Grace has been writing for magazines for over a decade, with stints at *The Times*, *Vogue* and *Glamour*, and has freelanced for *Sunday Times STYLE*, *American Vogue*, *Allure* and *Teen Vogue*.

Starting out in fashion journalism before switching to beauty, Grace added a new topic to her repertoire in 2012 when a stranger ploughed into her labia with a pair of surgical scissors and changed her life forever. And henceforth, like most mums, she struggled to keep every minor parenting victory and vaginal trauma to herself.

She lives in Sussex with her husband and her daughter.

This is her first book.

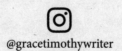

@gracetimothywriter

@gracetimothy

LOST
IN
MOTHER-
H◯◯D

LOST
IN
MOTHER-
H⬤⬤D

GRACE TIMOTHY

HarperCollins*Publishers*

HarperCollins*Publishers*
1 London Bridge Street
London SE1 9GF

www.harpercollins.co.uk

First published as *Mum Face* by HarperCollins*Publishers* 2018
This paperback edition published 2019

1 3 5 7 9 10 8 6 4 2

A catalogue record of this book is
available from the British Library

ISBN: 978-0-00-827870-0

Printed and bound in Great Britain by
CPI Group (UK) Ltd, Croydon, CR0 4YY

MIX
Paper from
responsible sources
FSC® C007454

This book is produced from independently certified FSC paper
to ensure responsible forest management

For more information visit: www.harpercollins.co.uk/green

This book is dedicated to my girl, of course. Kid, you made me as much as I made you, and the world is so much better with you in it. I love you. Thanks for your patience, your joyousness and your helpful notes. You're already wise and funny beyond your years. I'm excited about you, bubs – go get it.

CONTENTS

PROLOGUE

I attempt to sit still, to look as relaxed and open as possible, but I'm on one of those chairs that leans back on a bendy frame. You know the ones? That kind of plastic-looking blonde wood with a creamy-coloured leather cushion. I looked it up online after our session – it's from IKEA (obviously) and it's called 'Poang', which is Swedish for 'point'. As in, *what's the point?* I think people buy them as nursing chairs, too.

Well, I would have lost a nipple if I'd tried to breastfeed in this chair, let me tell you. My stomach muscles were shot to hell once I'd given birth and I'd have been about as steady on a rocking chair as a drunken eel. Plus, my vagina was so mashed up, the idea of grinding it back and forth on a beech veneer would have broken me for good. I definitely rocked in those early days, but it was more of the rocking-in-a-dark-corner type of move, deprived of sleep and a functioning pelvic floor. The sort you can do on completely immobile furniture or even the floor.

You have to be so cocky to make one of these chairs rock gently and comfortably, and not throw you off like a spooked horse. I am not cocky or relaxed in this scenario, and have to slam my feet down suddenly to steady myself. I'm aware it's made me look uneasy. One false move and you look like you can't handle it. This chair is basically a metaphor for motherhood and the predicament I find myself in now.

I am sitting here in a stranger's living room with no shoes or socks on. Bit weird. It's OK, I'm actually here for a nice bit of reflexology, with a birthday voucher from my mum and I'm finally getting round to using it six months later, on the day it expires. 'You deserve a bit of a treat, darling,' she'd told me at the time, 'You look a bit knackered.' *Weird way to kick me when I'm down,* I think, smiling through clenched teeth at the thought of trying to fit in this so-called treat, and of the new electric toothbrush I'd hinted at for three weeks. But my mum volunteered to babysit and now here I am on Pat's Poang, answering her questions about my medical history.

I'm an easy customer in this respect – no operations, no medications, no family history of diabetes. Uneventful pregnancy and straight-forward vaginal delivery. Couple of stitches, nothing to write home – or down on a form – about. I don't have so much as a high blood pressure or a tennis elbow, so we whizz through the checklist. *A nice little foot rub,* I think to myself, *Might be awkward when she finds the verruca I picked up at BabySwim, but otherwise, I'll just sit here, relax, be serene …* Then she says it:

'And how about your emotional wellbeing, how are you feeling right now?'

I smile, a smile I plaster on my face, which should say *I'm fine!* But usually makes people take a step back and ask, 'Are you sure?' from a safe distance. It's become my 'mum face' – the mask that covers up the underlying cocktail of anxiety and bewilderment which has been simmering since I gave birth nearly three years ago. But this time, it slips:

'I would say … well, I am maybe a bit anxious. Well, a lot. And most of the time, too.'

'Oh?' She doesn't seem surprised, 'And why's that?'

'Mainly because I love my daughter so much I'm terrified I'll lose her or fuck it all up for her. I don't think I was ready to have kids and I have literally no idea what I'll do when she starts nursery because I don't know who I am anymore without her.' This sounds much worse out loud than in my head and I think perhaps I've overdone it a bit. 'I mean, don't get me wrong, I love being a mum!' *Reel it back in. Don't call the Social, don't take her away!* 'But I find myself just bowling through the routine every day and then feel a bit joyless when she's gone to bed. Like, what's it all for? I mean, I really enjoy my job, but doing it makes me feel guilty, plus, I'm not sure I'm very good at it any more. Is she even having a nice time? I don't have much of a social life anymore; I don't really have many friends nearby. I don't really know what to say half the time. I've also lost my sex drive,' – I soundlessly mouth 'sex drive' rather than say it out loud – 'my body, my name even …' I pause – the massive digital clock on the wall flickers to 10.25 and breaks my flow. It's a beautiful autumnal day and I catch a glimpse of golden leaves and rolling hills outside as the Roman blind is blown away from the window for a second. It feels good sharing like this out of my family's earshot.

'So you feel it's changed you, Grace? Becoming a mother?'

One minute I was just me, doing my thing. I defined myself by my likes and dislikes, my desires, career and relationships. I did whatever I wanted to do. After years of body-image battles,

I finally felt like the agent of my own body and I'd grown to understand how it worked. No matter how far I travelled or how my life changed slightly, the constant was the familiarity of my own self. But a cursory New Year's shag before the takeaway curry arrived was enough to change my life forever. In that instant, I lost control of my body and mind as they were repurposed to grow a baby. My identity started to slide off me as hormones and then love infiltrated every thought and feeling. The colleagues, friends and even strangers who played a part in shaping and supporting my sense of self slipped away, work dwindled as every hour became a moment in my child's life. I felt like I had to fight twice as hard to have a voice. My confidence was knocked by the constant feedback from *everyone* and their suffocating deluge of opinions and anecdotes. I tried to fit in everywhere – old life, new life – and didn't fit in anywhere.

It doesn't matter how you come to motherhood – biologically, by adoption or surrogacy – it changes everything. You are now a MUM. What I experienced is an identity crisis which no social group, age, creed or race is immune to. It's something I've heard of in different forms from every mother I've ever met, an uncomfortable truth that belies the belief that being a mother is the most natural thing a woman could do. From the physical and emotional changes you encounter to the way your agenda and daily life is altered, your identity is constantly up for redefinition. '*I thought I was patient,*' I would think to myself, '*I thought I was bright …*' And you're expected to shelve these concerns because you don't matter anymore. Not compared to the baby, how you're working to help shape *her* identity.

My coat is folded over my lap and my fingers are burrowing through the pocket where a thread has come loose. I tug at it, pushing my fingertips through the ragged seam into the lining. This coat is enough of an answer to this question. I find a small, plastic toy fish floating around. Found Nemo, didn't I? That would obviously never have happened to me before I had a child. Nor would the crispy Wet Wipe I'm nudging aside. Nor the coat itself – a navy blue, knee-length puffa coat, waterproof, functional and covered in stains. You don't have a coat like this unless you're a mum or a shepherd.

In truth, I'm unrecognisable from the person I was just three or four years ago, before I got pregnant. If you'd told me back then that I'd be sitting here now deep in the Sussex countryside, wearing leggings that bag around the knees and pouring my heart out to a total stranger in a beige tunic, I would have called bullshit. Back then I was invincible and so sure of myself.

But here I am in this ugly chair, one finger now tangled in the lining of my mum-coat, mid identity crisis. I've lost sass and flirting, and about 65 per cent of my labia. I've lost perspective and 5,689 hours of sleep. I don't stride or strut now; I hurry and chivvy, usually weighed down by my child, umpteen bags or a scooter. The responsibility is weighing heavy too, for this person I love so intensely – I am her advocate, I am her carer, and I have to get it right. But can I ever be good enough, be the parent she so deserves and I am in no way qualified to be? And where am *I*, where is the confident person I was before? I am now the wife who blackmails her husband for lie-ins, who criticises the way he looks at his phone when his child is asking him a question. I'm the woman who drives around for hours on end if it'll help my kid nap, rather than face the screaming and ultimate failure of putting her in her cot and hoping for the best. I forget to turn up to things, I flake out on the nights out I used to live for, knowing the next day will be unbearable. I stand back from conversations with new people, no longer sure of how to introduce myself.

The simple bits of being a mum are obviously awesome – everyone knows how good it feels to hold your child, to laugh with them, to share their joy and see things afresh through their eyes. Even the more mundane bits can be an unexpected treat – it always surprises me how much I enjoy washing and drying her clothes, for example. I pick up the scrap of cardboard that holds the yoghurts together and tell my husband, 'Ah, we'll make something out of that'. I absolutely love being my child's mother; nothing has made me happier, or could ever make me happier than being her mother. Nobody could love her more.

And this kid – she is the most amazing child. If I can't excel at parenting this one, I'm seriously inadequate. *She* is incredible, the best thing ever. But the *stuff* is harder than anything I've ever endured. It's hard sharing the experience and responsibility with someone else who may not always agree with you, the loss of sex and intimacy with that person, the onslaught of self-doubt. It's hard to get through each day on so little sleep and then each night – hallucinating, nursing, arguing, worrying and begging for rest. I feel guilty when I'm not with her, guilty when I'm with her that I'm thinking about not being with her, or because we're watching too much TV. I'm always tired, always.

I've been policing myself, too – cautioning myself not to become *that* kind of mum or *that* kind of woman. No sugar, no soft play, no iPad, no tacky plastic shit, no chemicals … but also, like, super-relaxed and laid-back. My ambitions have been compromised, of course they have, but what's worse is that it bothers me. I'm also bad at work now, and when work's going well, I'm bad at being a mum. And I'm scared *every single day*, scared she'll die, that I'm doing it wrong, that I'm letting her down. I realise neither Pat nor I have said a word for a long time now.

'Soooo, will we do the foot rubbing bit now?' I ask eventually.

'If you want to, but we can just talk if you'd like?'

Uh oh, sounds like Pat might be moonlighting as a therapist here, I think. *Oh, I shouldn't have said anything.* When I'm not forthcoming, Pat places her pad down on the floor and reaches out to hold my hands in hers.

'I think you really need to invest in some space for yourself,' she goes on, 'Have you tried meditating? Book 15 minutes out to meditate, another 15 for a walk outside, just you. And I think you'd really benefit from some body work too – regular sessions with me and maybe some cranial osteopathy. You need to make time for yourself, Grace.'

I consider this. 'Do you have kids, Pat?'

'No.'

'Ah.'

PART I

THE THREAT

CHAPTER ONE

THE FIRST TRIMESTER/SHOCK

You just know when you first find out you're pregnant that having a baby is going to change everything. The obvious things like your day-to-day life, your financial status and your independence are hanging in the balance. Your home will quickly fill with plastic toys, the corners softened, the plugholes stuffed. Your body will be repurposed like a dodgy doer-upper on *Homes Under The Hammer*, which you might start watching because you'll suddenly be switching from working woman to stay-at-home mum, at least until the stitches heal, but probably for a year.

I was most worried about how becoming a mum would affect my identity, with which I'd only just felt comfortable at the age of 28. If work, marriage, friendships, your body and even your name are directly affected by this twist in the road, where will YOU end up? 'Just A Mum' and nothing else? Finding out I was pregnant felt like taking a pair of scissors to the threads which my future hung from, *snip-snip-snip* – I knew I would have to change and I didn't want to.

I know – this is not how books about child-bearing usually begin. They're all BLESSED to be with child, the fulfilment of a lifelong dream to be pregnant. Well, I could write that book, for the record. My love for my child is endless, boundless and unconditional. I love being her mother. But this book is not about my baby or my relationship with her. It's about saying, without caveat or excuse: being a mum is better than I'd ever imagined, harder than I thought possible and I am a completely different person now. I have gone through a transition at a rate that would make your eyes bleed.

If that's not enough and you're about to cast this book down in disgust and write me off as undeserving of the gift of childbirth, let me pre-empt some of the hard stuff with a little story. You're still getting to know me, after all, and this story is quite a good yardstick for measuring my kind side.

When I was 19, I saved up for months and months to go on a turtle-saving expedition. If you've seen that Attenborough documentary or *Moana* you'll know that turtles lay their eggs in the sand at the top of the beach and a baby turtle's instinct when it hatches is to scratch its way up through the sand then head for the sea, scuttling towards the light of the moon bouncing off the water, where it will swim away and presumably find its mum and live a long and fulfilling life. But, sadly, now there are hotels and traffic to confuse them, many will wander the wrong way and try crossing a road and die under the wheels of a car. Also, they are poached and made into soup.

So I selflessly left a summer of partying behind me at my peak party age, and started trawling the beaches of Grand Cayman at 5am every morning to check nests and help any little guys that had got stuck to crawl up through the sand and make it to their destiny, to fulfil their little turtle dreams. So when you're thinking, *JESUS, THIS GIRL IS BLOODY AWFUL TO*

HER HUSBAND/MUM/GYNAECOLOGIST, just remember the tiny turtles I saved and how nurturing and motherly I must be beneath all that bravado. Ahh, little tiny turtles, guys! What's cuter than that? God, I'm such a good person.

Before I became a vessel for my mother-in-law's third grand-child (if that wouldn't make a great slogan tee I don't know what would) I felt fairly sure of who I was. Actually, I never paused to think about it. I felt young first and foremost – endless possibil-ities stretched out ahead of me once I'd earned a bit more money and turned 30. A map of places I would one day visit, a menu of experimental haircuts, clothes that really lasted and a collection of house plants lay in wait. I was building up to all that and in the meantime I was a swearer, a drinker, very occasional smoker and when I went back to my parents' place, still an idle teenager, glued to their sofa because they had Sky and I wasn't yet adult enough to sort that out for myself.

By 28 you kind of know the sort of friend you are, the sort of girlfriend, the sort of daughter. You know what makes you tick, what you can and can't stomach, which drinks will make you blow chunks all over a car park and which will help you live your best life. You know how you handle work, stress, heartache and you know what kind of social being you are. But you prob-ably have no idea what kind of mother you'll be.

There was a lot of trial and error to make the 28-year-old me. A lot of hard work to take me from diligent intern to magazine staffer, then finally to this freelance career as a beauty writer, which was just taking off. I had fallen in love with my husband Rich at university and so we had grown up together and whittled 'young professional' identities side by side. Like most millennials,* we had lived with my parents for six months, and that's as hard as it got for us.

We saved up and bought a tiny flat in Brighton once we were both working, and continued to save for sofas and TVs and maybe a holiday one day. Thanks to Rich's unshakeably stoic and calm personality, I never had to work very much at being a girlfriend or wife, because it was the easiest gig in the world, but I was very aware of – and grateful for – our dynamic as partners. I remember reading an article in a bridal magazine when we were first engaged which asked, 'What kind of bride will you be?' and I remember thinking, *just like, me … but in a wedding dress?* It hadn't affected either of us at all, getting married. I hadn't even changed my name. During the week I was still a hard-working, single-minded writer for women's magazines, and at the weekend I was a semi-retired party girl. I had just discovered karaoke and how adept I was at Cher's greatest hits. I hadn't encountered loss or redundancy or impotence – nothing that could throw me off-course for even a second. I was surrounded by brilliant, funny women all the time, who were just as selfish as me. There wasn't a baby amongst us, just a working week punctuated by red wine, books, boxsets, shopping for olives and sex with my husband. There was no ill that couldn't be remedied with a cocktail, a cheese sandwich and at worse, a cigarette. I was solid and robust.

---

* Am I a millennial? I suspect I'm too old. It's loosely defined as one who reaches early adulthood in the 21st century, but I would argue I haven't really reached adulthood yet.

Then one New Year's Day, my husband thumbed in a softie just before the curry arrived, and somehow that was all it took to derail this well thought-out life. We hadn't even had sex in a purposeful, deliberate way, really. Having been together for six years already we didn't do it as often as we used to, and on New Year's Day I was always overcome by a combination of hangover guilt and the need for fresh starts to announce that we would be doing it more often that year. We would make it a priority; it would be our New Year's resolution to shag plentifully. And so every year, despite not wanting to, we would have sex, because to not have sex would set the tone for the year. But this perfunctory two-minute act was all it took to get those robust Yorkshire sperm into my reticent, slightly uptight eggs and lo, I was up the stick. Getting pregnant was the biggest curveball I'd ever been thrown. It was the ultimate kick-you-in-the-gut moment for a control freak like me, especially as I assumed I was infertile on account of the chlamydia.*

Too much? If you're feeling like you already know more than is necessary about the workings of my genitals, I urge you to continue regardless. (Except you, Dad. If you're reading this, chlamydia is a rare but very beautiful orchid. Don't read the footnote, 'kay?) Think of it as an endurance test of sorts. I'm not sure what the reward is for enduring multiple descriptions of my innards, but still.

---

* Just to clear something up (as that nice GP did with my chlamydia, thankfully) – I contracted this symptom-less disease when I was in my late teens. My boyfriend at the time, a lovely Catholic boy from the countryside, who waited patiently for months before having sex, was secretly riddled.

I blame motherhood for the need to over-share. I never used to discuss my vagina with anyone who wasn't directly involved with it, and that was generally confined to my gynaecologist and my husband, and before that, a brief but distinguished list of men in their late teens/early 20s. And most of them didn't discuss it per se, as much as compliment it or suggest it be better groomed.

But the minute my vagina was ripped open by a crowning head in a room of eight strangers, it became public property and my number-one topic of conversation. I took back control by talking about it to everyone, presumably so they'd get a fair idea of what it was like before they inevitably saw it. It's possible I need therapy. Anyway, buckle up, there's more to come. You'll be able to draw a very accurate diagram of my labia by Chapter 7, and I urge you to do so.

Wait, why are there TWO lines?

Let me take you back to the moment the story really began. It's 9.15am on 24 January 2012, and I'm at home in Hove, sitting on the toilet, staring down at the knickers looped around my knees. Tears are quietly pooling in the gusset. I have just seen two blue lines darken purposefully on a pregnancy test, where I'd have preferred just the one, and maybe a thumbs-up emoji. Because two lines mean, yeh, you are all kinds of pregnant. You've basically AirBNB'ed your womb; another human being is setting up camp in your innards. Your vagina is about to be split in two, then chopped up like mincemeat.

It was not the news I had hoped for when I planned to fit a quick pregnancy test in between breakfast and the start of my working day, writing about – ironically – whether it's ever OK to ask a woman when she's going to have kids, for the *Huffington Post*. It was off-topic for me, but since our wedding in 2010 it was all anyone asked me and it had really started pissing me off. I mean, sure, on paper, my husband and I were all set for the childbearing years to begin. But the assumption that as a married woman the next logical step would be motherhood irked me. I am a fully practising feminist so I'm not into the yokes forced upon our sex. But also I was still keen to prioritise spontaneous holidays and sleep. Oh, and my career. And I just didn't fancy it.

Then I realised I hadn't had a period since 2011, so when I popped out to get the paper and live yoghurt (in case it was thrush delaying my menstruation) I added a pregnancy test to the basket. There I was, midway through furiously tapping out this angry argument that 'when are you having kids?' was an entirely inappropriate question when I saw that the answer from me would be, IN ABOUT NINE MONTHS ACTUALLY.

My first instinct was to go back in time and nuke that errant sperm, ripping its microscopic little head off and dousing the remains with a shot of spermicide. I know, I know – I seem like such a maternal soul, why on earth would I not want to embrace this little miracle?

The truth is I enjoyed being an autonomous, self-obsessed, one-blue-line kind of person. I liked who I was. I liked our tiny flat full of sharp corners and bottles of rum. I liked my husband. I even liked my body. I didn't want all that to change. Plus, I was about to start a new job which I had spent the past seven years working my butt off to bag (often for free): acting beauty editor at *Glamour*, a part-time gig so I could also start writing a book. It felt like I'd finally got to where I wanted to be.

Just the week before I'd been sitting in the pub with a group of girlfriends slagging off people with kids for invading our favourite brunch bar – the buggies skinning your ankles and the thoughtless amount of noise and space-invading stuff these women came with. The general gist was: mums are selfish and obsessed with their kids and lose all reason and ambition when they give birth. They moan and stop dyeing their hair. They don't have sex anymore. They live vicariously through their kids, letting their own lives slip from the radar. They lose the will to engage with the world and crusade for what they believe in, unless it was #FreeTheNipple or banning junkies from parks.

I was fine with concealing my nipples and would a Brighton park even be a proper Brighton park if it didn't offer a grassy knoll up to a junkie once in a while? I couldn't join this gang now, swallow my words about not letting prams on commuter trains. Also, imagine not being able to have a sneaky smoke when you felt like it. What would I do with my right hand when there was a bottle in the left?! I did another test. Still pregnant. *Fuck.*

How can you become a mum and not lose your sense of self? I considered the examples of motherhood I had to go by. Kirstie Alley in *Look Who's Talking*. Diane Keaton in *Baby Boom*. She had given up a kickass career to make apple sauce. APPLE SAUCE? I hate apple sauce. And how about *Three Men and a Baby*? What drove the mum to leave her baby at that weirdly massive loft apartment and flee when she could have stayed and asked Tom Selleck about his moustache? Plus, it took THREE men to keep said baby alive, by the way. It wasn't just something I'd gleaned from Touchstone Pictures, though. A school friend of mine had got married and had a baby all before I'd finished university. The friend I'd danced up against on smoky dance floors, sneaking a Volvic bottle of vodka from my mouth to hers had a son, an actual kid that was hers. All I'd gleaned when I popped in before returning to the smoky dance floors was that she was hoovering all the time and seemed … dazed. Happy, but not like before. Different. Like a body-snatched kind of different. Not a happy I could understand because it revolved around nappies and a crying baby. Of course, it was love, but I was too self-involved to recognise that.

Wiping my pee-soaked fingers on a wedge of loo roll, I wistfully looked over at our wonky airer, where I'd layered T-shirts, thongs and a pair of leather trousers to dry. I was nostalgic for the moments before I found out I was pregnant and just chucked clothes about in ignorant bliss. *Oh my God, I'll never be able to have sex again,* I realised. *Mums don't really have sex unless they absolutely have to, oh God!* I kept checking the skin on my belly – the freckle, the barbell through my belly button. I didn't want the freckle I'd looked down on forever to stretch, and no doubt the piercing would just come shooting out at some point, like a bullet. I'd have to give up my job, move house, shop in Mothercare. Suddenly all the framework for my independence was wobbling, teetering.

I cried hysterically, and wandered into our tiny living room, readying myself to call the baby daddy – currently at work – and tell him he'd made me pregnant. For a moment, I was the only person in the whole world who knew our lives had changed forever.

When he picked up, I gasped and gulped and snorted.

'I NEED YOU TO COME HOME!' I eventually shouted into my BlackBerry, snot and spit peppering the screen. 'NOW.'

Silence his end.

'Are you OK?' he asked at last, his voice naïve, full of hope.

'NO! I'm not very … well.' I answer. *I can't tell him I'm pregnant over the phone, knowing he has an hour's commute to survive,* I think to myself, *wait 'til he's home.*

'Fuck, you're pregnant, aren't you?'

'Yes.'

'FUCK.'

The baby daddy

If this was a romcom, Rich would have rushed in and we'd sit together (in a much bigger room in a bijou flat, lit by twinkly fairy lights). He would smile as I cried fresh pretty-faced, snot-free tears, which were all down to shock and could be easily mopped up. I think my hair would be up in an artful topknot, tendrils cascading around my forlorn but very beautiful face. He would rub my back while telling me all the cute things we'd enjoy doing with our baby, his boyish excitement spelt out by a grin and sparkling, earnest eyes. He'd sell me a lifestyle of scooting to the park, baking cookies, swimming in lakes, handing every full nappy to him, until my crying turns to laughter and we smile at each other. This little wobble would be tied up nicely so nobody would worry, everyone would know I do really want my baby – of course I do – and a happy ending is around the corner. Nobody wants to think of an unwanted child! That's a horrible proposition! It's possible a Beach Boys' song would accompany the end of the scene as we are holding each other, as trepidation turns to joy. *It's all going to be fine!*

Instead we perch on the edge of our new sofa, he puts his head in his hands and neither of us talks until the sun has set so low someone gets up to switch on a light.

I met Rich several times before I met-met him, because, I argue now, I wasn't ready for the onslaught of love and feelings. I was helping out with the Mr Nottingham University pageant, which he entered, and had a boyfriend at the time, so I wasn't primed to see him as a prospective baby daddy. His special talent was to down two bottles of wine in under a minute, and then set his balls on fire. He also sang 'Wonderful Tonight' while stark-bollock naked, but I think I was in the loo at the time. I was introduced to him again at a party a month later, where he'd just had his head shaved for charity, but again I don't remember it – not ready. I needed to fuck around a bit longer and flirt with my friends' brothers, etc. When I did properly meet him, he annoyed and interested me, which is of course a fatal mix. He was one of four irascibly arrogant, attractive freshers who turned up late to Rag orientation, just as I was halfway through my speech as a committee member. I balled them out for it but took note of his blue eyes, cool glasses and the ridiculous way he was wearing two T-shirts at once. And while I publicly raged against arrogance, it basically turned me on (I was 20 years old, nowadays I just rage). Even though he was pretty direct, I could never tell whether he was joking or not. He was really funny, acerbic, incredibly rude and a showman, and I dug it. But once I'd made the first move (drunkenly standing on his feet, thinking I was playing footsy, and then just shoving my tongue in his mouth), it turned out he was also deliciously kind, sweet, clever and sane. Definitely not my type – I liked them dark, swarthy and mean – but it was a nice change. He was so level-headed and patient, which was comforting to a highly neurotic crackpot like me.

He's from Barnsley and had only left the UK for UK-extensions, like Faliraki and Kavos. His ambition had been to open a cocktail bar OR fight fire (mainly with the view to nailing chicks), with no ambitions to go to university. His teachers thought otherwise because he was really clever, but it wasn't until a friend's father suffered a massive stroke that he decided to study physiotherapy at university, thinking he could be pivotal in the rehab of people like his friend's dad. I know – whatta guy. Nearly 11 years later that's what he does – helps people learn to walk again. He's basically a good man with a questionable sense of humour.

We are the stereotypes of our regions in the flesh – I'm every bit the southerner his parents feared I would be (precious, fussy, always cold), and he's every bit the northerner my parents hoped he'd be (calm, stoic, economically sensible).

He's got lips like Tom Hardy and despite the fact he has mousy-brown hair, is convinced he's blond. He's got a dead tooth up front where he flipped over the railings inside a double decker bus with a beer bottle between his teeth. He has a broad but soft Yorkshire accent, and swears in a southern accent – a hint that perhaps he didn't swear at all before he moved down here. He's always very good at everything, even if it's his first time. From table tennis and playing the ukulele to useful things like building a shed and card tricks. He's a bit tight; slightly sloppy when drunk and when he buys something he has to check its price remains the same online in the weeks afterwards.

He's kind, quietly and understatedly. Kids love him. Everyone loves him.

I'd had boyfriends before we met at 20, but I'd never felt this genuinely worshipped, and it made for a heady end to my second year at uni. One time we staggered back from a night out and there was a sign on the old fridge which my landlord had dumped in the front garden, saying to 'look inside'. He had filled the whole thing with cheese, massive blocks bought from the cash and carry, like gold bullion in a safe. It was the most romantic thing anyone had ever done for me. When I graduated, I continued to go up to visit, and when he graduated, the following summer, he moved down to Chichester to my parents' house. When we both got jobs – his as a physio and mine as a writer – we moved to Brighton, where we've been ever since. He is still the anchor that keeps me sane but also laughing until I pee, and although he is nearly a whole year younger than me, he is always the more emotionally robust of the two of us. I often look to him for a measure of a situation, when I don't know what to think. So the fact that he wasn't jumping at the news was making me even more nervous. *It's his baby too, and he's more worried than me.*

Proper weepy

The next day, after dreaming about growing phantom babies that were actually kittens, I wondered if maybe the problem was that my husband is so laid-back and rarely visibly excited (I blame his northern upbringing) that I just hadn't been buoyed along yet? *Maybe I need to seek out the joy, absorb it like osmosis from someone who will be really excited.* So I hopped on the train to see my mum. I placed the two positive pregnancy tests on the table, and predictably enough she squealed with joy. I was banking on her reaction making me feel happy but the bitter tears came again, the inexplicable sadness. I couldn't say those words – I AM PREGNANT – without sobbing.

'I've saved all your Sylvanians, darling!' she says, as if this would steady my nerves.

She realised the escalating price of toys wasn't the problem, and held me for what seemed like hours.

I dodged calls from friends, came off Twitter and I put on my out-of-office. I told Rich I wanted to be sure how I felt about it before I dealt with how other people felt about it. Deep down, I think I wanted the option to back out of the pregnancy, but also because in telling people, *they* would start seeing me differently too. I didn't want people to start vying for my job or friends to discard me on the pregnant pile. I shut myself away and didn't deal with it at all. Until my body forced me to deal with it.

I'm just like Kate Middleton

I was back at my mum's a few days later when I was suddenly punched in the throat by a wave of nausea, which never let up. I crawled into bed and there I stayed.

'Oof. Oooooof, ooooooof. Oof,' was all I could say. Almost the French for egg, interestingly, seeing as it was an oeuf implanting itself in my womb and causing me to feel like I could fill a stadium with my hot, sour vomit.

The early symptoms of pregnancy are the first hint that you are slipping from your own narrative. You hand over your body and mind to your baby and to everyone who has an opinion on how you should look and feel. For me, it felt like my body was turning against me, like the priority was already switching from me to my baby, who as yet was just a cluster of cells. My body changed in a flash; I had lost control already. As I was at my mum's when this tsunami hit, there I stayed. It was insane! My every cell vibrated with the need to vom and that sappy taste sat on my tongue like an oyster. My mum wedged halved Cheerios between my cracked lips so I wasn't starving her grandchild, but otherwise I didn't eat and I would spend up to 10 minutes trying to swallow a single mouthful of water.

It wasn't just the mornings either – it rolled through my body 24 hours a day, waking me from sleep. I couldn't escape it. Lying down, sitting up – it was all like riding a rollercoaster – and I couldn't read or focus on the TV to distract me.

My acute sense of smell meant that I knew Rich was entering the house before I heard him. His aftershave, his breath, a cigarette he'd walked past that morning – it was all burning the hairs out of my nose, making me hate him. Hate him! This prick with a penchant for pickled onion Monster Munch was clearly out to piss me off.

'YOU HAD A KFC, DIDN'T YOU? ADMIT IT! YOU SELFISH ARSEHOLE!'

Weirdly, he stopped asking me how I was feeling about the baby around then. And with my mum hovering like a nervous nurse, wringing her hands and counting Cheerios, it was easy to avoid the conversation altogether. I think he assumed I would be dead soon, anyway.

I felt so weak and so sad now; the need to stay in bed and sleep was overwhelming every other thought. *This is what depression feels like*, I thought one morning as I considered changing my pyjama bottoms but instead rolled over, a fresh wave of nausea drowning me under its sour wash. I had experienced brief pockets of depression in my teens, so I knew the familiar heaviness, the consistently tear-filled throat. Looking back, I definitely suffered from antenatal depression. It felt bottomless and constant.

It was pulling me under and away from decisive action, stopping me from making a plan to surface again and change. Suggesting anything as definitive as an abortion at this point felt too deliberate and I was wrung out, not capable of lifting my head from the pillow. I definitely thought about it. I was adamant I did not want to be a mother. And the craziest thing? I couldn't tell anyone how I felt. Because the first thing a mother is expected to be is loving and grateful.

When I read about postnatal depression I felt a bell ringing – *I've already had that,* I thought, *that's how I felt as soon as I found out.* Now I go to the PANDAS Foundation UK website and see that as many as one in 10 women will be depressed in pregnancy. As a clinically recognised diagnosis it is only about 20 years old, perhaps because the effects of pregnancy can make the most robust of women feel shit. The painful tits, the dizziness and breathlessness, the nausea, the realisation that your only source of support is a total bellend who can't ball his own socks let alone care for a baby. But it can also be down to a hormone imbalance: levels of the hormones oestrogen and progesterone increase during pregnancy, which usually results in that 'bloom' women are supposed to enjoy as they gestate. But according to PANDAS, sometimes the placenta doesn't produce enough progesterone, which can lead to chronic anxiety, incessant crying, lack of energy, isolation … yes, yes, yes, and hell, yes. Had I known this, I could have asked for help. But I assumed it was all part and parcel of me being such a bad potential mother.

Every outcome seemed wrought with sadness – having the baby, not having the baby – as I sunk lower and lower.

After years of routine smears finding those pre-cancerous cells you've got to have fished out from your cervix, I had a gynaecologist. It sounds grand, doesn't it? – 'MY GYNAECOLOGIST' – but actually, it was the grim reality of having the suspect cells. I no longer needed to be referred by my GP, I was a regular at the salon-de-speculum. Anyway, when my mum eventually decided I wasn't peeing often enough, she took it upon herself to call this gynaecologist (did I mention she was also my mum's? YEP, we have the SAME gynaecologist) to ask her advice.

'Bring her into the hospital this afternoon – I've got a clinic just outside the antenatal unit, I'll squeeze her in.'

Perks of having a terrifying vagina, guys! Straight in! I was pulled from my bed, whimpering, refusing to put on clothes.

'Could you just breathe through your nose?' I asked my mum, tsking her appalling breath, as she drove me to the hospital, my neck craning out of the window like a dog.

'Yes, you're definitely pregnant, Grace, congrats!' the gynaecologist crowed, as the transvaginal scan revealed a tiny, peanut-sized lump lying in my womb. 'And there's only one baby, great! I was worried about twins or triplets with the way you're feeling,' she qualified, cheerily.

'Yay!' I whispered. I cried quietly as she ran through all the brilliant things about this baby – the scan was showing it to be the perfect size, the placenta was on track, it would have a September birth, which is excellent … *I mean, what fucking brilliant news, September you say? I'm so pleased that this foetus will most likely excel at school because it'll be old for its year. Marvellous. But now what about if it was born in 2020? Because I think that might work better, actually?* When I feebly mumbled I was scared for my vagina, she assured me that the vagina could be stitched up like any other battered body part – 'it might actually be *better* afterwards', she said, winking at my husband.

Then my test results came back and it turned out my ketones – the acid that remains when your body burns through its own fat because it has little else to burn for energy – were really high. Like, anorexic-in-hospital-for-a-feeding-tube high. So they decided to admit me, put me on a drip and try medication for the nausea.

I was officially diagnosed with Hyperemesis Gravidarum (HG), which once Kate Middleton was diagnosed in 2012 became all the rage. Back then, I'd never heard of it. It's a condition affecting 1 per cent of women suffering with sickness in pregnancy, according to Pregnancy Sickness Support. Symptoms include hardcore pregnancy sickness which could actually harm you and the baby, if left untreated. So if you took pregnancy sickness and gave it some crack and some Red Bull and said, go to town on that woman's gag reflex, bitch, that's it. The causes are unclear, but I suspected it was thanks at least in part to the fact I wasn't that up for having a baby right now.

I felt like a massive failure, taking the drugs. Mainly because I hadn't considered the risk to the baby until my mum had piped up. But also because my body – according to the doctor

– needed the drugs. If I didn't get a handle on the nausea, the pregnancy could end anyway.

It looked and felt as though I was dying. The nausea might last the entire nine months, said the gynaecologist, but they could make my body a bit more hospitable for the baby. *Wait, why is nobody seeing what a terrible idea this is and suggesting it would be safer to end the whole debacle? I have very narrow hips.* I silently begged them to find a medical reason we had to abort, using just my eyes. Which of course didn't work. I wanted to talk to Rich, but he was ushered out with my mum so I could rest. It was as if he'd faded away from this picture altogether – it was just me being poked and prodded for signs of life.

When my mum came in to collect me the next day I stared at the TV, answering her questions with a grunt or a sigh. I was so cross with everyone who was *meant* to be on my side but had already sided with this new baby, who nobody had even met yet. I had been hospitalised! I had a cannula sticking out of my hand because the acid coursing through my veins would other- wise kill me! *I am SO ill! Why is everyone congratulating me?* I cried some more.

Back at home, my mum helped me shower and propped me up in her bed, facing the TV, just as she had done the last time I had puked Gallo rosé wine all over my own bed 10 years before. The drip had definitely taken the edge off and the medi- cation was dulling the nausea so that rather than feeling violently sick with every breath, I could almost picture myself eating dry toast one day without heaving.

The best thing that'll ever happen to you?

When you're pregnant and feel ill-equipped, you say things like 'What if I drop it or slip over and squash it?' to your partner or your parents and they'll hush you with platitudes, as if all those outcomes are impossible. Nobody's going to suggest an abortion, no matter how scared you are. They might secretly be thinking, wow, she should NOT be having a baby, but they'll never say it. Even my mum, who had delighted in the goriest details of my birth for the past 28 years, suddenly shut up shop on that particular theme, and just kept telling me that becoming a mother was the best thing she'd ever done.

That's a pretty big statement, I thought. I appreciated the sentiment, of course – I was that baby that outdid every other experience she'd had to date – but … really? I mean, it was better than falling in love with my dad? Better than riding a motorbike in full leathers? She'd lived through some pretty incredible moments – first female prime minister, first woman in space, first computer, the advent of the NutriBullet … She'd nailed a dozen different careers, had accomplished so much. She'd seen friends beat cancer, she'd watched the Berlin Wall tumble down, she'd met Katharine Hepburn and Ingrid Bergman. She'd been a punk, a speed freak, an artist, an island-hopper – surely there must have been some serious highs in amongst all that hedonism? Before you had to ditch the Marlboro Reds and black coffee and rely on me – a jelly-mouthed baby with colic – for your kicks? Having a baby was the best? I hadn't done nearly enough of all the other stuff yet, could it really eclipse all the other stuff I'd planned to do?

I realised I couldn't have a straight chat with her about this – she was too deeply invested already, and she was One of Them

– a mum. She couldn't give objective or impartial advice on this. It felt like she was just full of massive Hallmark lies. And more lies: I was seriously ill but nobody would openly discuss the prognosis. I felt sure Rich and my mum were shaking their heads in the next room, wondering how they would raise this child together when I had died in labour.

Now, usually when I'd gone through something a bit shocking – an especially bad commute where there had been no free seats and I'd had to witness someone vomit into their briefcase, for example – I'd unwind with a little drink. I liked to sit on the windowsill in our bathroom, with a big glass of wine and very occasionally, a cigarette. I'd flop from there directly down into the bath and give myself a massive head rush from the combination of smoke and hot water (I'm actually a bit of a pussy when it comes to both of those two indulgences – I once passed out after half a Benson & Hedges at school). Clearly, cigarettes are a big no-no during pregnancy, but booze? Rich was adamant it was stupid to abstain altogether.

'Have a glass,' he said. 'It'll relax you and I've been reading up – it won't hurt the baby.'

But the real kicker was that my body disagreed. The minute a bottle was opened I was overcome with the urge to throw up. The smell was unbearable. As was the smell of tea and coffee. And food.

So it seemed my body was actually siding with the baby now, too. It was coming round to the idea of growing a healthy child. Which was hard when all my comforts – reflexology, aromatherapy, sex – were being stripped from me. I got very dramatic when my mum suggested a hot bath might not be a great idea.

'I read that if it's too hot it could harm the baby. Plus the pH of your vagina is sensitive so bubble bath might irritate it, which is no good because you shouldn't really take antibiotics.'

'GOD, MUM! Is there anything I *can* do? Can I take a shit in peace or WILL IT HURT THE BLOODY BABY?!'

'Just don't push too hard, darling!' she called after me.

I tried to slam the bathroom door and cursed its slow-close safety fixtures. Great for not smashing a kid's fingers if you have one, not so much if it's you who wants to throw a tantrum.

Neither my mum nor Rich would acknowledge the logistical flaws in this new life plan, either. Whenever I mentioned worries about how I'd continue to work and therefore pay the mortgage, my mum would say something like, 'It'll be fine,' or 'Well, there's never a good time!' *If there's never a good time, why the fuck do people ever have babies at all?* I wondered. I'm pretty sure if I'd been suggesting buying a second house, they'd have some objections. But that was safely off the table because no mortgage advisor would be able to sanction such a thing. A similarly expensive investment by way of a baby? Shockingly, nobody's doing risk assessment on that.

So I called my uncle. He is a very wise man who has self-helped himself into a pretty solid mental state, and is always called upon by every generation to give advice on money, work, relationships and dry wall. It's weird because he's never had kids, has never married and he works for himself, but I think it's the fact he always seems happy and his irrepressible can-do attitude that makes him the ultimate agony uncle. *You want to travel? Do it. You want to sell up and live on a barge? Why not?* And so it was decided he would help this reluctant mother-to-be reconcile her Beyoncé-styled feminist stance on womanhood with impending motherhood.

'I don't see how this is going to change everything if you don't want it to,' said THE MAN WITH NO KIDS AND NO UTERUS. 'I mean, you decide how you want to play it, it's your kid. You and Rich are smart enough to make it work. Look how many women carry on working and socialising?' He basically told me to Lean In. It was what I needed to hear.

'I don't even know if you have to move out of the flat – kids are small for ages, right? For now, just call your boss, sooner rather than later, and see what she says. If she's adamant you can't do the job, you'll know and you can make a different plan. But it's really her call, so find out and you'll have all the facts.'

He was right, and in my head this handed at least an aspect of the decision over my future to someone else, which I liked the idea of. Yes, my boss could decide if the idea of parenthood was viable for us.

Rich finally made his way into an empty room and we lay together holding hands. He told me if this wasn't the right time for us to have a baby we could discuss … the alternatives. Just like that, the unmentionable had almost been mentioned. There was something about laying it out like that, making it real, giving me the very real chance to say, I don't want this, which set me free. It was all it took to make me breathe again. I thought about it. If I didn't have a baby it would mean an easier ride at work, that we could plough on unimpeded in many ways. But for some reason, even though this pregnancy had seemed like the worst shock, it was softening around me. It seemed less of a doomed situation. I felt scared, and when had that ever stopped me from doing anything? I mean, apart from waxing my bikini line. I wasn't ready to throw a baby shower and buy a cot, but I was getting closer to accepting pregnancy, which was easy since I couldn't see or feel it yet. I asked Rich what he wanted, and realised he just looked truly knackered. He shrugged and said he felt it wasn't the best time, and he was worried about my career.

'You've worked so hard to get here to this point, and I know it's hard to risk all that.'

'So if I wasn't worried, if I could carry on working, would you want this baby?'

'I think there are so many questions though – how would we make it work? But ultimately, I guess we just would.'

He's very good, isn't he? Didn't overtly lay the entire decision at my feet but didn't commit to his own opinions either. He was just supportive and patient.

'What about partying with your friends and your career, and what about the flat?'

'Well, those things will be there whenever we decide to have kids, won't they?'

I decided to try on a different hat for a moment. I'd never delivered this as good news; I'd rung him bawling my head off, after all.

'Fuck it,' I said, 'Let's have a baby.'

'OK, bubs.'

He said later it was like a switch had been flicked inside me, some kind of maternal ignition or something. The mood had changed and he went with it.

So I decided to get my ducks in a row, starting with work. I plumped for an email because 1. I am chicken shit 2. I still couldn't talk coherently, and knew for sure heaving over the phone was not going to help my cause. I've always hated that a phone call gives you the opportunity to talk in the wrong place, to stumble over your words. My boss replied – congratulations, I still want you for the job, we'll see how it goes.

Oh! So it's fine then. Huh.

It felt as if the final concerns had been washed away by this woman who couldn't see any harm in me doing both – pregnancy and a job – so now I really had the chance to mould this situation to suit us. It felt like she was all, you can handle both – you can do it. It didn't *have* to be the end of life as we knew it.

I carried on feeling sick, hopeful that I'd feel better at 12 weeks because I'd heard this was quite likely. I was counting down the days, either sweating under a blanket on my mum's sofa or sleeping. Usually sleeping.

When I was 10 weeks pregnant, I had a bleed. Nothing dramatic but a definite red bloom in the gusset, sticky and ominous. I called the antenatal unit at the hospital and was finally put through to a midwife who was eating her lunch at her desk.

'Nothing you can do, love,' was her brusque summation. 'It might be that you're miscarrying but we don't do scans this early on, so you'll know at your 12-week scan. If you lose a lot of blood, call 999.' And that was it. I might be miscarrying, I might not. It could all be gone in the next 12 hours if the blood continued to come and the little clot of cells fell out of me.

I felt that hot prickling around my hairline, a signal that my body was preparing to fight or flee. *Interesting,* I thought, *I'm definitely not relieved. I am worried. I don't want to miscarry, actually.* The contrary brain had turned. The fragility of this baby came shrieking into my brain, and I felt protective. An hour or so later, I was reading the copy of *What To Expect When You're Expecting,* which my mum had popped on my bedside table weeks ago and had sat there gathering dust ever since. I let them talk to me as if I was a happy, expectant mother, as if this was all part of the plan and I was now excitedly entering the second trimester. Suddenly, when it was suggested in real terms of life and death – that this wasn't a fait accompli I simply had to come round to – I could feel something different. By not worrying about my identity, my career or my relationship, something else broke through … An instinct? I'd be the first to call bullshit on that – I hate the idea that we're biologically structured to make decisions that will make us good mothers – but just as the antenatal depression and sickness had felt out of my control, so too this new acceptance and sense of calm came without a rational thought.

I just knew I wouldn't miscarry. I knew this baby would come and although I wasn't sure what would follow, I looked forward to that moment. Of course, I could very easily have miscarried and I'm astounded I didn't. I am not a doctor, I know nothing. But the awful chemical reaction that was making me feel so hopeless and frightened seemed to slow, the hormones settled, and I was sure. I know, it sounds like I was properly crazy, and I was, but that's hormones for you. Or at least, I hope it was the hormones. Otherwise I was/am properly crazy. I began to look beyond the immediate moment, just a little bit past it to the 12-week scan.

Oh, and by the way: I hate turtles. I hated getting up at 4.30am for our beach treks, I hated the smell when I had to dig down to help the little cretins reach the top, I hated the fact that you'd think they were dead, lodged in the sandy cavern, but then they'd suddenly flip around and spray sand in your face. I went on the trip to drink rum, meet guys and party with my friend, who had coerced me into including this turtle crusade in our itinerary so we had something to put on our CVs. I remember thinking, if these tiny creatures that everyone finds so cute are lost on me, I'm clearly NOT a maternal person in any way. But, remember: HORMONES.

CHAPTER TWO

THE SECOND TRIMESTER/DENIAL

OK, nothing's going to change. We are in control. We will be FINE. *A baby is just us plus one.*

A midwife calls me 'mum'

The 12-week scan arrived and we sat alongside other women at various stages of pregnancy in a corridor outside the ultrasound room. We were back in Chichester because I hadn't yet mustered the energy to leave my mum's and go back to Brighton, it's where Rich worked and my gynaecologist was right there. Without making any hard and fast decisions about how it would work when I was due to give birth, we had opted to register at this hospital, an hour's drive from our flat.

A colleague of Rich's waved at us – Rich, my mum and me – from across the room, his wife bulging at the seams, and thus our cover was blown. But it didn't worry me now that we had a plan of sorts. Plus, we were a party of three – four, if you counted unborn foetus – so we stood out a bit. My dad was due to come but I wasn't sure if it would be another transvaginal scan or not. Transvaginal is so not my dad's thing, weirdly.

I still had trouble equating everything I felt with an actual baby – I felt like I had been hijacked, but possibly by some kind of government-funded scheme to secretly investigate chlamydia scar tissue in 28-year-old women. Not a bouncing baby. But the nausea had finally chilled out to a low-level feeling of crap, which I could thankfully eat through, so I was feeling better at any rate.

The midwife bellowed my name into the waiting room – cool, officially and publicly pregnant then, thanks, love. I was convinced that since I felt so inadequately equipped to become a mother everyone waiting probably thought I was too. I had this feeling that they all thought I was a young teen mum despite the fact that I definitely looked like a 28-year-old mum.

We went in and the nurse signalled to the bed while looking over my NHS-issued purple book of notes.

'Now, if Mum could just jump up on the bed, and pop your jeans down, please.' She was still looking at her notes, and so I wondered why on earth she would want my mum to pull her jeans down. Mum looked back at me with the same confusion, until Rich edged me towards the table. And just like that, this woman changed my name.

I felt like saying, *Oh, actually, we've decided nothing's going to change? Yeh, so just call me Grace. Grace is GOOD, thanks.*

I really like my name. Grace is easy and singular. It's what my parents chose and I love them very much. And so I love Timothy as well – it's pretty much the only thing I have in common with my six half-siblings. It's what I took into new schools as a little one, it's the thing I still have from those days. In fact, other than a brief phase around eight or nine when I'd asked my parents to call me Olivia Graceland, I had always been called Grace. I didn't qualify for nicknames really, because it's not something that needed shortening and I probably didn't have any strong enough traits to mark with a cool moniker. I didn't even change my surname when I got married. As a journalist you work so hard to get it known, handing out business cards whenever possible, repeating it over and over so all and sundry know who to call back for another internship. I was by no means well known, but if I rocked up with another name all of a sudden, wouldn't I be someone else? Wouldn't I lose a key bit of myself, and potentially not be remembered? Rich had made a big deal of the 'emotional emasculation' in his wedding speech, but he was actually behind me on this. We hadn't quite got to the whole what-will-our-kid-be-called? convo, and I had already decided I didn't mind a bit if she or he was a Holmes. But anyway, I spent a bit of time thinking about it and explaining it, and now this stranger had changed my name in one swift move. I was officially 'Mum', despite the fact my child was a mere cluster of cells. I don't even know why I'm defending this whole debacle actually – it's my name, I want to keep it! End of!

Being referred to and introduced as 'Baby's Mum' is as reductive as it gets. I mean, I am used to being introduced as something to place me in someone's mind – so-and-so's assistant, The Intern, Rich's wife, Blonde Grace (at uni, I was one of two Graces, Boobs Grace and Blonde Grace) – but being called 'Mum' was a bit like being renamed.

I know it sounds like I was worried about losing my cool, but in all honesty, I was never cool. Anyone who mewls, 'I used to work at *Vogue*!' four years after they've left and relies on a knock-off designer handbag to help her be taken seriously in her industry isn't genuinely cool or really that OK with her choices. BUT, I did have a sort of mask of cool perfected. I had some of the right clothes, I had focused on constructing this career that would take me to cool places where I would sweat profusely and wonder if I ever pronounced anything correctly. It was definitely a façade and I'm guessing the imposter syndrome was what was causing my upper lip to be perennially moist. It was a relief to go freelance and only have to maintain over email. But I did believe the last vestiges of anything resembling cool would trickle out of my vagina with the baby. Or, ideally, be delicately lifted from my insides by the surgeon who was performing the C-section I was fantasising about. Because I'd then forever be known as MUM.

And is it any wonder?! When do we fetishise or even celebrate motherhood in our vocabulary? When do we use the words in praise? In fact, my generation have advanced the field by adding the prefix 'mum' to things that are really rubbish, to really drive their naffness home. For example, 'You're such a mum' – you nag, you worry, you piss everyone off, you big fat bore. 'You're so mumsy' – you're dowdy and dumpy and nobody fancies you. 'Mom jeans' – the ugliest fucking jeans known to man. They make your vagina look like a big ass and your ass look like a big vagina. FACT. 'Mommy porn' – 50 Shades of grammatical errors and submission-based sex. Yuck. I'll take me some non-parent-related porn, thank you. 'Mum hair' – a really crap bob.* 'Mum face' – haggard, grey, tired-looking

---

* Although, to be fair, I think we're reclaiming that one with the ubiquitous topknot and young people seem to love those. The rattier the better. So maybe we can still turn this one around.

complexion. Probably teary. 'Yummy Mummy' – mum who makes a bit of an effort, which for me always had a whiff of the Readers' Wives about them.

Sometimes 'mothering' someone can be kind of nice, but it's 100 per cent sexless and non-exciting, and tends to be a way of gently pointing out you're treating someone like a baby. Rather than being fabulous and dazzling, you're patronising and basically suffocating another person.

So then, mums are tedious, past it and irreparably uncool. You are JUST A MUM. Nothing more than that, even though the 'just' suggests you ought to be. I sneered at the idea it would be the hardest job in the world, but fully believed it would be the most boring one. Once we've started to make progress on making BITCH and CUNT unacceptable, we're going to have to explain 'mum' isn't really such a hot diss. It's just another way of reducing women, of dismissing and degrading them. And it totally worked on me.

Mums are parochial and stuck in the 80s – presumably because that's where we've banished our own mums to. They're subsumed by domestic drudgery, hoovering in the background of the real narrative, ready to cook or wipe a bum. They are overcome with tiredness and the shame of having no sexual appeal whatsoever. In fact, they have sex only to have more babies, surely?

My mum the wild child

It's weird that I was so convinced by this depressing idea of motherhood, when my own mum wasn't really like that. It turns out that although she and my dad had been trying for a baby for a couple of weeks when she got pregnant she still had the same pangs as me, worried about the changes she would be going through. Maybe more so, given that her own parents had split up when she was a child and her mum had never really recovered, dying of a broken heart when she was just 58, all her birds having flown the nest. My mum, in comparison, was a wild child. She didn't so much dabble in drugs as body-slam herself full force into bags of speed and weed. She had a lot of sex with a lot of people. When she met my dad she was a theatre stage manager, working late into the night, partying hard and sleeping until the matinée started the whole cycle again the next day.

'What did you do on Sundays?' I once asked. She couldn't remember there being any Sundays.

Then she met my Dad. She was in love. So in love that she – the least maternal person ever to walk the earth, she says – married him (even though he had six children) and decided to have a baby.

When she got pregnant her sisters laughed and her dad shook his head gravely. She'd been babysitting my baby cousin for a full 30 minutes when he'd rolled off the bed and cracked his head open on the floor. It was a terrifying prospect. But she quit the fags and coffee, got really fat and eventually bore me into the world.

She wasn't like the other mums. She didn't bake or sew or knit. She dyed her hair pink. I never thought of her as 'mumsy'. She and my dad were considered 'a bit showbiz' by my friends' parents, I think because they had a lot of gay friends and said 'cunt' a lot. They threw parties, were out every weekend and she was a force to be reckoned with – a strident feminist and purveyor of crude jokes in a village of doctors and accountants, all of whom voted Tory and sailed every weekend.

She never 'settled' in motherhood, she still thought everything could be bigger and better. With her on the PTA the school fete suddenly went from a little jumble sale to a gala for over 3,000 people with celebrity guests, hot-air balloon rides and a remote broadcast from the local radio station.

Mumness

So it was weird that I was really preoccupied with an image of mums cleaning floors and loading the washing machine – great work, advertising industry! Drinking insipid tea in front of daytime television with a worried look on your face. I think I got this from *Neighbours* or *Coronation Street*. I was also pain-fully aware I'd need to learn how to make gravy. That seemed important somehow.* 'MUM' was the refrain moaned by pre-teen boys in grass-stained football shorts or precocious girls with gappy teeth and pigtails. It was a word always whined or howled in my head.

Of course, it ended up being the most loved sound in my universe – when my kid first mumbled 'mama' it was like I'd discovered who I most wanted to be right there. So in the right hands, when it was *her* saying it, it was the most beautiful sound, like liquid gold. To be fair, she once called me a slut

---

* I mean, I actually met the OXO Mum. I met her! She also played my dad's wife on TV. And to be totally honest off-screen I didn't even know she had kids. She had a filthy laugh, a killer body and lots of mascara on. Everybody stared at her, she was magnetic.

(having heard it on the radio, mind – nothing to do with me) and even that sounded bloody lovely. If I reduce it right down to its fundamental parts, it's love: motherhood is love. So the name really has bugger-all importance. But back to pregnant me, who had no idea that would be the case.

I wasn't even on Instagram back then. I didn't have that group of women saying, 'Look, you can wear neons and you can get shit pierced and take your kid to gigs! Look at our snazzy backpacks and our gin!' Without social media, your tribe is whatever you have in front of you. And I was working in an industry where having a baby could end you unless you pretend like it didn't happen. A baby in a sling was about as likely to win me work as suddenly admitting I had shagged the boss. Actually, less so, because most magazines wouldn't want me to write about my experience of childbearing.

But then the cold jelly was dolloped onto my stomach, that weird barcode reader was pushed down hard and we heard the swooshing 'thud-thud-thud' of a heartbeat. I looked at Rich – *Oh my God, are those tears in his eyes?! Is he … is he crying?!* – and missed the baby coming into view. When I looked back at the screen it looked like a little puppet. It had the hiccups, according to the sonographer, and we watched as it bounced off its soft bed, limbs flailing like a little Thunderbird. It didn't look biological at all, it was mechanical and cloudy, like really bad TV.

'But I can't feel it,' I said, completely unable to see this image on the screen as a snapshot of my insides. Not like with a trans-vaginal scan, where you can feel the probe knocking your ovaries like a piñata. It still wasn't a baby there on the screen, but it definitely looked like something which might grow into one. Rich was transfixed and I felt bad that I wasn't bonding with the squiggly little creature that could have been anywhere. It was still sexless in my head, without an identity. But I took the picture they printed and tried to see Rich and I in the image. There was my long chin at any rate, but the long hooked nose looked like a little old man's. I stared at the picture long and hard to try and see our future – *this is our kid*, I thought, *this is our kid. This is Rich's kid! I love Rich and this is his child, inside me. This is my very own kid* … It didn't really work, but I've never been very good at pep talks.

Then we left and went back to real life, away from this crazy world where we gazed into my belly, and pressed on with the present.

I nearly puke on Anna Wintour

When you're pregnant you can deal in these diametric opposites quite comfortably as the future is all hypothetical and you can't imagine not being in control of your own destiny. Moving on from the fear of a baby changing everything, I had resolved that it would change nothing. *I don't want to go to soft play or parks, so I just won't!* I thought, making a mental list of the things I didn't like about childcare and so would just not indulge. I practised full-scale denial, thanks to the advice of mostly childless people and from reading books by women who had nannies, even though I knew we'd never be able to afford one.

And continuing as if nothing was going to change was actually completely possible during my second trimester, as my energy returned and the sickness calmed down. My belly started growing but the bump was still very much of IBS-bloating proportions and sometimes barely appeared at all. I hadn't bought a stitch of maternity wear, I was working out the perfect anti-nausea routine in readiness for a return to work, and I was about to prove my theories and capabilities in the most sane way I thought possible: attending Fashion Week. Unfortunately, it would instead be the moment I narrowly missed vomiting on Anna Wintour.

To give you a bit of background information, when I left university I went straight to *The Times* as a fashion intern. From day 1 at the newspaper, I was hooked. I had a string of badly paid internships and quickly realised that to make the knock-backs and hard graft worthwhile I would need to become fiercely ambitious.

I eventually got a job at *Vogue* based solely on the fact that my boss at *The Times* gave me a good reference, and that I spoke Italian (which actually was not true).

Then a job as an actual WRITER came up at *Glamour*, where I stayed until I'd amassed enough experience to go it alone as a freelance beauty writer. I compiled a list of dream titles I'd try to write for, and at the very top was *American Vogue*.

So when Style.com – the sister site from the same publisher – asked me to report backstage at London Fashion Week the week I was diagnosed with Hyperemesis Gravidarum, I was like, obviously, yes. At the time they were THE authority on the shows, I'd be mad to turn it down. And if I stepped aside for even one season I'd be quickly replaced by someone who *wasn't* inconveniently breeding.

It was just a shame I felt so sick.

I decided to keep my 'condition' top secret from those around me.

The first show was at the top of a very high, very glass build-ing, and as I'd over-planned I arrived about an hour early. I stepped out of the elevator, into a vast warehouse-style room, with all the action focused in one corner of rails and pop-up hairdressing stations. I took in the view and as I swayed aboard my ridiculous 4-inch heels, my mouth began to froth. *NOT NOW, NOT NOW!* I reached for a cracker and scoffed it down like the Cookie Monster, spraying flecks all around me. Then the lift pinged again and out stepped La Wintour. Maker and breaker of careers. Editor-in-chief of the magazine at the top of my wishlist, the doyenne of cut-throat fashion-ism. On any other day, had I not left the top button of my jeans undone and just sprayed water biscuit down my front, I would have approached her. I knew it could be a terrible idea, for sure – she had a brutal way of dismissing people, I'd heard – but her daughter had interned with me at *Vogue* and I'd met her again on a trip not long after and she was lovely, warm and generous. I had an opener. I wanted it so badly. I wasn't scared, I was ballsy.

I'll just go up to her and be all, HEY, ANNA! I know your daughter! Super-casual, just one professional to another. So I straightened my shirt, smoothed my hair down. I got ready to make the ultimate career move.

But instead? I burped. Like, really loudly. Loud enough that the people to the rear of her entourage cloud turned around. I turned around too, as if to ask, WHO WAS THAT?! Then I lurched forward, stumbled backwards, and then hid behind a rail of clothes for the next 40 minutes, dry heaving.

Well, this is new, I thought. Not the dry heaving at work – we've all done the morning-after-the-Christmas-party-retch –

but the complete lack of control and professionalism in the face of a potentially big career moment. Being pregnant was definitely jamming my work mode and it scared me – what if, no matter how much I try to stay the same, it would actually be impossible? It was so frustrating and terrifying to feel the bit of me that got my mortgage paid and fulfilled my ambitions was under fire.

I managed to write the reports and by staying away from the other beauty editors who would have known what was up when they smelt my acrid breath and the fact that I wasn't stealing the models' croissants, nobody was any the wiser. And I decided that once the morning sickness had completely stopped, I'd be able to continue unchanged. The fact is, I'd been in the room with Anna and co., I was still allowed in. I just needed to rein in the impulse to vomit.

We need a new nest

OK, so I was still adamant that nothing had to change. But one thing really did – where we lived. Yes, quite a big thing, actually. The flat that we'd scrimped and saved for, and made our mark on by way of two floating shelves and a new catch on the shower door, had to go. It had been perfect, pre-fertilised-egg – a living room with giant sofas that doubled as a large dormitory for friends to crash out in, and a windowsill over the tub, for stacking candles, books and the occasional bathtime sandwich.

The summer before I'd got up the stick, we decided to put the flat on the market because we thought it might be time to splash out on a garden of our own. Somewhere to drink coffee on a Sunday morning, maybe a box room I could make my office now that I worked from home. It sold at the first viewing (and that shower catch made us £15,000 – snap!) but we couldn't find anything nice we could actually afford. We dawdled and ummed and ahhed, because we were under zero pressure – *so what if the buyer pulls out, we don't HAVE to move, and we'll just get another buyer.*

But at the end of February, as I entered my eighth week of pregnancy from my mum's sofa in Chichester, our buyer finally threatened to pull out if we didn't vacate within four weeks. Rich started to rush over to Brighton after work to check out other flats and back to me in Chichester each evening to endure my rants about his breath. One evening he arrived back from our flat, another bag of my clothes slung over his back, and slumped down next to me on the sofa. I didn't mention his personal stank because he looked so broken. I'd basically been ignoring him for a month and hadn't noticed how the commuting and lack of support was getting to him.

'Look, we need a plan. Nothing new is coming up, we can't afford anything suitable in Brighton. We have to be realistic.'

Nonononononononono!

'I think we ought to start looking outside of Brighton. We'll get more for our money. And I won't have to commute as far, which means I'll be back before the baby goes to bed. Brighton is not going to work for us, not right now.'

He'd said it. It was out there. Our life *was* going to change. But there was a caveat – *NOT RIGHT NOW*. Once we'd saved a bit of money, maybe we would be able to go back to Brighton, to a proper house. This wasn't forever, this was for now.

'And I think the most sensible choice is right here, because I won't be far from work, you won't be far from the hospital and your parents will be nearby to help out.'

Fuuuuuuuuuuuuuck! I'd no longer be the city girl, living a stone's throw from her favourite bar, the beach and an ATM machine. I'd be back to where I started, back to bad phone signals, no nightclubs and a lot of fields. Back to socialising with my mum and wider family without having a cool flat and glamorous job to jet back to afterwards. Back to feeling gawky and isolated and frustrated.

'OK,' I say, in the tiniest voice, hoping he might not hear and we can just pretend this hasn't happened. I have no fight in me, and I'm pleased that he seems buoyed by this decision at least. I can deal with the finer details later. At least I wouldn't have to meet another set of midwives either, or try to navigate a new set of roundabouts, my bête noir as a driver.

My mum was delighted, Rich was grim, and I was escaping it all on Rightmove. It had replaced ASOS as my favourite virtual shopping basket. I was already changing, *OH GOD, NO! Ooh, but wait, look, a double garage!*

I was supposed to start my job in six weeks' time, and we would have to have moved before that. And actually, there was a whole bunch of small houses – HOUSES – for the amount of money we'd saved for a one-bed garden flat in Hove. They were mostly new builds – small Tardis houses with boxy rooms and a manicured lawn of fake grass. Then behind door number four was a 122-year-old tiny cottage, with pink roses and a rambling garden full of wild flowers. We both had to duck as we entered and quickly calculated we'd have to ditch both of our sofas. The owners had a baby, so a metre from the main bedroom on a floor that inexplicably sloped and creaked was a tiny box room, barely big enough for a single bed, but already decked out with a cot and shelves of stuffed toys. My mum warned us off it – 'It's old! It probably has damp! And what about the sloping floors?!' – and Rich scraped the skin off his scalp by head-butting the doorframe, but I was in love.

Rich was less keen.

'There's no room for our sofas. And what about the floating shelves, where will they go?'

'It's bigger than a flat though, isn't it? And there's a garden.'

'Well, we wouldn't be able to have the Wii out. It would have to go in a box or something.'

'Um, OK. Or we could plug it in upstairs in the loft? Hey, you could have your own game room, bubs!'

'Hmm … But what about my bar? Where would I put my bar?'

DEEP BREATH.

'Rich, I'm not sure we can discount a house on the sole fact that your bar – which maaaaybe isn't the priority when we have a baby on the way – doesn't fit in. AMIRIGHT?'

'Fuck.'

'I know, dude. But … well, why don't you build a shed in the garden and put your bar in there? It could be proper bar, then, couldn't it?!'

'Hmm …'

For Rich it was the realisation that we were settling down, becoming a family, but true to form, it took him 24 hours before he was immersed in the positives, excited about building a shed with a bar in the garden, and as we stood outside Boots with a bag of breath mints (attempting to continue to abate nausea), the estate agent called to say we'd had our offer accepted and would hopefully exchange in June. The next day I drove back to Hove with my mum, stopping en route to dry heave onto the hard shoulder, and put down a deposit on the first flat I viewed for rent, based purely on the fact that it was near the station. Currently occupied by a woman with cats, it smelled like cats.

It would be the stopgap between our old life and new, a quick commute to London until I could commute no more and would be hoisted into our new cottage, ready to hang up lines of tiny baby-sized washing and start puréeing apple sauce. I could take the stack of magazines we used as a coffee table and our collection of novelty shot glasses, it could still feel like home. Sure, we'd have to pay rent and a mortgage for two months, but we would otherwise be homeless. It was all coming together and I had two major projects to occupy the part of my brain that would have otherwise freaked out about the baby. It was still half a year away – no biggie. I helped pack up our flat (well, I lay on the bathroom floor, shouting instructions to Rich), and although I felt those glum feelings returning – we were essentially packing up our youth and independence into those boxes – I focused on the immediate future: an exciting new job and a slightly briefer walk to the station in the morning.

The fabulous thing about moving while pregnant – which we would do twice – was that nobody wanted me to do anything. I went a bit peaky, fetching sandwiches for lunch, and all the removal men stopped what they were doing to pep talk me into sitting down. Rich rolled his eyes as one of them picked me up and put me on the one remaining chair they'd left in the middle of the now-empty living room. Sweet.

Rich and I went to a swanky fish restaurant that night.

'This is the new us, bubs – OK, so maybe no to nightclubs, but this is really nice, isn't it? We'll go to nice restaurants and widen our culinary horizons! We'll be fine, actually, won't we?'

He nodded, as he poked the skeleton of his sea bass, wondering which bits he could actually eat.

Bloated yet professional

Finally, we were installed in our new flat and the day arrived – I was to begin my new job at *Glamour* on a shoot day, interviewing the model Lily Cole while my beauty boss styled her and directed the shots. And it was like I'd never left. There was no mention of babies or morning sickness or the future. I was singing showtunes with the manicurist, wheedling Lily's favourite lipstick out of her when all she wanted to discuss was her work for Greenpeace, and fingering a rail of glitzy threads I could never afford. I WAS BACK. It was familiar, it was comforting, and it was work.

Nobody knew I was pregnant, of course, and I wondered if the information about my expectancy would be announced officially or would drip-feed down from the higher echelons. It's the latter, and one by one, startled staffers came by my desk when my boss was out to hiss, *Is it true?!* One wasn't convinced, even when I showed her the shape of my belly under the massive shirt I was wearing.

'Yeh, but your boobs haven't got any bigger, though, have they? They're still really tiny.'

Always a pleasure chatting with that one.

I called on an old colleague from *Vogue* one lunchtime and she helped me navigate Topshop's maternity section. I was finally kitted out and my belly was no longer covered in livid red indents from my savage jeans.

Work was a true sanctuary, and even as my bump swelled and became more noticeable, the team mostly ignored it as per my request and I was not once sidelined. In fact, when I was five months pregnant, my boss assigned me two trips: one to Paris to interview Natalie Portman and just before that, one to LA to launch a new shampoo. I know that sounds ridiculous, but yes, we were flying to LA in order to sit around a table in a conference room and discuss a new shampoo. I said yes to both without hesitation, calling Virgin on my boss's request to check I would be OK to fly. All was approved and I was off to LA!

On the morning I was due to fly to LA, I woke up at 5am, worrying I'd miss the alarm, so when it went off I sprung out of bed and started busying around the bags. Rich lifted his head sleepily, reached for his glasses and stared at me.

'Oh God, what?' My hands immediately jump to my belly, thinking it's probably ballooned overnight.

'Have you … spilt something? On your … tits?'

I looked down at my white T-shirt. Two little yellow splodges sat right where my nipples nudge the cloth.

'What the fuck?!'

It was like a watermark on silk, a ring of yellow syrup. Actually it was more like pus.

I ran into the bathroom, squeezed my nipples and all of this thick yellow mucus dribbled out. Of course, now I know this is a natural process – it's the colostrum gathering ready for your baby, and actually it would have been worthwhile trying to 'harvest' some of this nectar. But I was horrified. Pus tits?!

Other than the fact I had to stuff my bra with the hotel's complimentary cotton pads every morning, LA was GREAT. Without Rich or my mum there, I could completely deny the pregnancy was taking hold of me. I was in a fabulous hotel with fabulous people, none of whom were parents, and I didn't really even look that pregnant. I didn't get jet lag, which was awesome, and by not drinking I felt pretty fresh, actually. My belly had grown while I had been in LA – possibly because of the travel-related water retention, but either way, it got bigger.

I still didn't *feel* pregnant, just bloated, but I got slightly panicky about the changes. No going back now, it was happening.

Weeks later, I was in Paris.

Natalie Portman: [passes a beautiful hand over my belly, which is bigger because I just ate a burger while waiting for her] 'Oh, my! How far along are you?'

Me: 'I think, like, about five months? But I'm not really sure actually, because I *think* I got pregnant on New Year's Day, but there's of course every chance it was before that and my dates are all messed up because I can't really remember when my last period was, you know? I mean, it's possible I just got that wrong, but that's all the doctors seem to be bothered about and I don't know when it was, I really don't. Plus, my husband and I weren't together for Christmas so we obviously hadn't really had sex between, like, 15 December and 1 January, that's two whole weeks! So yes, I'm not really sure.'

Natalie Portman: '… OK!'

And that was the last time *Glamour* sent me to interview a celebrity.

The gender reveal

You get two scans as standard during the second trimester, and at the 20-week scan I actually began to accept this was happening. We had decided to find out the sex of the baby at this scan. I'd been trying to look for signs that it would be a girl – three magpies, SCORE – and was actually pretty desperate not to find out she was a boy. Why? Because the only way I could get my head around having a kid was to imagine it would be like reliving my childhood, which I really enjoyed first time around. And if I had a boy, that would have been my last comforting lie to myself shot to shit.

'We don't look for the absence of a penis, now, we can usually see labial folds when it's a girl,' the midwife explains, as she presses the ultrasound into my guts.

But as we pretended only to care that the baby was healthy and well-formed, I yelped when the midwife announced:

'There's a vagina. I think. Labial folds. I think that is a vagina.' The baby kept crossing her legs – modest.

'Don't go buying everything in pink, now – this isn't a definitive answer,' cautioned the midwife, but still: A GIRL. And then she said, 'And here is your daughter's face.'

I felt a connection, at least with the concept of what was inside me being a baby. My daughter. Not some weird stomach bug or an alien creature I had no affinity with whatsoever. It was my daughter. She had lost the hooked nose and chin, and looked quite like a baby now, although I still couldn't feel the movements we saw inside me before. But there it was – I was going to have a daughter. She would be a girl and then a woman.

Rich and I agreed to keep the sex to ourselves. I was gagging to tell everyone, but he wanted to keep something back to surprise our families with so I agreed. I mean, I told my mum, my best friend, all my colleagues and a woman at the bank, but otherwise, it was absolutely a secret.

The nest is a nest for VERMIN

Things with our stop-gap flat started to go quite wrong as spring turned to summer. The line of woodlice marching across our kitchen doubled then trebled and eventually became an infestation. The landlord was all, 'Oh yeh, they're so annoying, aren't they? Hey ho!' I couldn't stand on them because they looked like they might be a bit crunchy so I spent hours every day scooping them up using Rich's driving licence, which I kept by the back door for this purpose.

The flush stopped working in the toilet, and the boiler cut out every other day. It was always cold and our clothes never dried.

Then one day I started to feel really ill while I was waiting for my train home. Sick, shivery, aching all over, like I was either going to puke, shit or die. I called Rich, who drove to meet my train at the station and took me home, where he put me to bed.

'It feels so cold,' I moaned as I fell into a fitful sleep. The next morning my throat was sore, my nose ached and I was breathless. Mum suggested I spend a few days with her so she could keep an eye on me while Rich was working. Rich and I went to throw a few things in a bag and discovered every single pair of shoes in the bottom of our wardrobe was covered in a thick coating of green mould. Rich pulled the wardrobe out of its recess and it turned out the whole of the wardrobe's back was green, too, with a swirling nucleus of thick white fur. That's when I realised our bed was damp, not cold, and the floor felt wet and greasy underfoot. He began stuffing salvageable stuff into bin liners, organising the stuff we'd need to decamp to my mum's again, and I watched him becoming a dad before my very eyes.

I was furious. Now, I probably always would have done so but what was interesting is how I kept referring to the unborn baby rather than myself as implicated in this gross situation. I got all my ducks in order first, calling the Environment Agency for advice on how to report this and how to handle our land-lord. Then I itemised the cost of everything that had been ruined – furniture, clothes, the bed, mattress, shoes, bags – so I could provide a clear invoice to offset against our security deposit and the next two months rent, since I was NOT going to be spending a moment longer in that hell hole. Finally, I got him on the phone.

'This is frankly untenable, and for the sake of my unborn child, I will not live here a day longer,' I concluded. 'I AM WITH CHILD!'

Well, this is interesting, I thought to myself, *it seems my maternal instinct is kicking in. Either that or I'm just trying to guilt him into giving us more money.* But it was the first time I had balled someone out for threatening the wellbeing of my kid.

So while we waited to move into our new home and our rental flat was being deep-cleaned, I was back at my mum's and she was nursing me through a fresh bout of morning sickness, but I was still adamant: *I will not lose myself, I will be different.*

I will remain ambitious, capable and when it comes, this baby will fit in around us, it'll do what we want to do. I just need to get my body back, and then? Back to normal for us. Even my mum backed me up.

'We just went out for dinner with you, you know, once I was upright again.' She winced at the memory but quickly continued, 'I mean, you just slept in your pram while we had dinner with friends, went to parties – you simply came with us. I went to Annie Nightingale's flat once and shaved half my head.'

This buoyed me. Rich and I agreed to dine out as soon as the baby arrived. None of this 'baby bubble', lying around in pyjamas for weeks on end, watching *Lorraine*. We'd get out there, get amongst it. We wouldn't have a single takeaway or frozen ready meal, and we would not get a microwave. Our new house would be a party house, always full of guests. We'd simply be US with a plus one.

To prove just how unchanged I was, I got dolled up and went to the *GLAMOUR* Women of the Year Awards.

'You don't have to come,' my boss explained. 'We totally get that all the standing around and the late night might be too much.'

'No, no, I'll be there!' I said, perhaps too enthusiastically.

I could still party, get my hair done, wear a dress that wasn't even from the maternity-tent section. Well, until 9pm, when the caterers cleared the plates, forcing me to stop minesweeping the leftover canapés, and I got a bit weepy in the queue for the toilets. As I was helped into a cab, I felt tired, a bit sick and very, VERY pregnant.

CHAPTER THREE

THE THIRD TRIMESTER/ACCEPTANCE

There's no denying it now – I'm huge. I'm fully repurposed. It's damned obvious there's a baby on its way. I'm a MUM and everyone knows it …

I was under the distinct impression that a baby gestated for nine months. There was that film starring Hugh Grant, wasn't there? And everyone says 'nine months' a lot, like it's the absolute maximum time you'll be pregnant for. But as I counted backwards on my fingers to the moment we *think* Rich impregnated me, I realise nine months is up and I'm still gestating. I ask the midwife, *Look, babe, are we nearly done here? Has someone made a cock-up with the calculations? Because I'm pretty sure we should be entering the labour phase now.* And she explained it was more like 40 weeks. THAT'S 10 MONTHS. More lies.

The grim realities of the final trimester – stretch marks, piles, breathlessness, aching joints – make it impossible to ignore the changes. Your body is totally foreign, you're staring down the coming weeks of what feels like the end of your career, and of course, the birth. The brain changes again – you must nest,

clean, furnish your home with the buggies, cots and digital ther-
mometers, all of which suddenly seem full of potential hazards,
each decision weightier than before. Your priorities are already
shifting. Your old self can still be heard – *Don't do it, don't do it!
Remember, we're not going to change!* – but it's all you can do not
to bulk buy nappies and dribble bibs. It was then I started talking about myself in the past tense a lot.

Growing a grandchild

The other thing that was worrying me a bit was the ownership
of the baby. Namely, the two grandmothers awaiting THEIR
new baby. I was fiercely independent and actually very selfish
with my time. But suddenly it wasn't about me anymore. HOLD
UP, WHAT?! There was a lot of talk about them not making
plans around our due date, so they could be there (*UM, unlikely!
You are strictly NFI to this cervical hoedown and that's a definite*). Then there were the various debates over who we would
spend Christmas with, from both sides. Now there was a child
added to the mix, I could no longer decide for myself where
we'd go and for how long – we were merely there to present her
to either side. It was the first encroachment on my selfishness,
I think. And I realised I was about to bring something to the
table that everyone wanted a piece of: BABY.*

'Why don't we do Christmas alone, just the three of us?'
I suggested to Rich when his mum first enquired, even though
I was still a whole month away from even *having* the baby.

---

* Not '*the* baby', you'll note because when you're pregnant, most healthcare
professionals drop the 'the'. It's just 'BABY'. Like Cher or Madonna.

'We can't do that!' He was clearly up for sharing. Typical youngest-of-three. 'I want her to be around her cousins and her grandparents. Christmases should be huge for her!'

I sulked.

I'd read somewhere that it was wise to lock everyone out for the first two weeks, and I agreed this was a sensible idea, based solely on the fact I don't like lots of people around and I planned on bingeing on series 4–6 of *Dexter*. But nobody agreed. My mother-in-law said she'd never heard of such a thing, and my mum refused to return her key. And now I get it – it's *their* grandchild – but at the time, I was just thinking of ME. *I do not want a house full of people when I've just given birth! I want time to adjust away from judging eyes, I want time to suss it all out and see if I develop postnatal depression before I have to think about entertaining guests. What, will I breastfeed and then make a bloody pot of tea for everyone?! Hoover when I should be SEEING TO THE NEEDS OF MY NEWBORN BABY?!*

But from then on it would be a battle of wills between me and the elders, who felt they had part-ownership of the baby. Not just in terms of the time they would claim, but also in terms of furnishings, apparently. Who will buy the pram, who will knit a blanket, who will provide second-hand monitors that already smell like electrical fires? My mum had already offered to buy us a new cot and changing station as a house-warming gift, and I'd agreed happily when I saw how much the bloody things cost. But then it was a bunfight in reverse. A car seat, baby bath and Moses basket were delivered within weeks of each other. I dumped them all in the shed in a fit of pique. If shopping was the only joy I'd get while my haemorrhoids were raging, I'd bloody well do it myself. You know, once the baby had arrived so as not to tempt fate, or whatever. Plus, we'd kept our mouths shut about what sex the baby would be, and it was killing my mother-in-law.

'But how will we know what colour to buy for it?'

'I mean, blue, pink, does it matter? Neither colour is going to harm the child, whatever its sex.'

'Well, you can't put a baby boy in pink, though, can you?'

OK. Deep breath.

'Well, what about grey? That's neutral, isn't it?'

'GREY?! You can't put a baby in grey!'

We dropped the subject but my mother-in-law later sent down a parcel of hand-knitted baby blankets, all in grey. And every grey babygro she could find. And it turns out they're quite hard to come by in Mothercare. So that made me cry, and also wonder if she wasn't actually trying to take control at all, but that my mad hormones had made me a bit paranoid.

My body is somebody else's temple

By the time I got to 28 weeks, I was bigger than anyone would have expected and there was definitely no denying it anymore. I heaved myself up onto the bus to work, sweating, huffing and puffing just taking the lift to the office. Eventually, my editor took me aside to tell me I could work from home if The Time comes sooner than we'd expected. And she was right. I kept on keeping on, thighs chaffing, bump propelling Londoners into oncoming traffic, but eventually I had to admit it: I was too massive to do the commute anymore. Enough. In July I agreed to work from home until the baby was born.

I started to think that the Victorian model of confinement wasn't such a terrible idea after all.

At that time I started going out a lot less, a sort of self-enforced confinement. I needed people to properly acknowledge that what was going on with my body was wholly peculiar. A break with life might be helpful, or at the very least an admission that it's very odd rather than everyone constantly poo-pooing your anxiety attacks because 'this is the most natural thing in the world'. That just makes people who don't find it natural feel crap. Pregnancy felt so unnatural, so utterly alien to me. It's no less shocking for its regularity. Everything felt different.

I want to look back and think, *I was a warrior*. I want to encourage other women to carry on being kickass while they gestate their kids. I'm not into any form of reverting back to Victorian-style womanhood. But I did a lot of reclining, swooning and weeping. Hell, if you're going to indulge in some naval-gazing at any point in your life, you might as well wait until that naval is swelling to epic proportions.

Meanwhile, Rich was getting a bit … chatty. I sensed he was getting nervous. He didn't ask how I was feeling a lot, or watch me with concern, he just kept asking incessantly, 'Do you fancy a wine yet, then? Or maybe some sex?' as if those were the markers of me being the same person still. As it happened I couldn't muster any enthusiasm for alcohol because it made me feel even sicker, and my sexual appetite had trebled because of my now-huge vagina, so again, nothing to persuade him all was unchanged. All the blood was rushing down there, presumably in readiness for the stretch of its life, but that also meant that it was sensitive as hell and I could basically get off just by wearing the right jeans. Going sofa shopping was way more fun than it should have been, and emergency stops were my new favourite car manoeuvre. I was a massive vagina with legs, basically. It did mean that sometimes when I went to the loo, the pee would spring up like a fountain rather than down into the bowl, but otherwise: good.

Rich was watching my body do some pretty weird shit, too. Despite the fact that I'd been slopping various oils across my bump for the past eight months (thanks to the dire warning from my mum that if I didn't I'd be 'riddled' with stretch marks), with two weeks to go, the piercing through my belly button which I'd removed months before grew a red forked-tongue out of the top and then a map of red threads snaking out of the bottom. A week later I had more red lines on either side of my belly button, and within days there was a tube map of livid scratches covering my entire stomach. Some of them sprang beads of blood as my skin started to break over the shape of the baby. I felt like it was only a matter of time before my skin would peel back and my stomach would burst. I still had a couple of weeks to go, when little spots began to crop up within the widest lines, followed by a rash that crept down my thighs and across my chest. It felt like my skin was on fire, it was so itchy. I went to the doctor, convinced I was about to explode, and he diagnosed something called PEP – Polymorphic Eruption of Pregnancy – which is an inflammation of the stretch marks. Nothing I could do or take, of course, because when you're pregnant, there's bugger all you CAN do or take. I tried icing it but nothing worked to calm the itch, and so I went up a whole new level of crazy.

I had been DUPED – I had done all the oiling and slathering I was told to do, despite the fact it felt horrible, and I had still got stretch marks so bad that they had their own acronym. I used to scream, 'BIO OIL!' as I dug my nails into my stomach when the urge to itch was overwhelming.

I only felt comfortable standing in the freezer aisle in Sainsbury's. I had to remain alert – if the sales team were aware I was loitering for too long they might think my enormous bump was actually a stash of petit pois stuffed up my dress, and strip search me. And while the walking vagina wasn't completely averse to that, I didn't want to have my Nectar card taken off me. In amongst the potato waffles and Cornettos I could peacefully waddle along, lunging to separate my thighs from each other as I went. I had a trolley to hold onto and a freezer to lean against – life was good. *Maybe I could give birth in here,* I thought, the idea of a warm pool making me wince.

Massive vagina aside, I was not enjoying this tail-end of pregnancy, which was clever of the pregnancy gods (who I assume are chaired by Heidi Murkoff, author of *What to Expect When You're Expecting*) because it meant I'd gone from fairly reluctant to give birth to actually thinking anything would be better than pregnancy. Maybe I'd even have an orgasmic birth,* I'd be that bloody happy to get things underway. Birth meant the end of PEP, the end of all the chafing and sweating and bleeding and gasping. I'd sleep again, pee normally again, maybe

---

* This is an actual thing and there's a book on it. Some women apparently get aroused to the point of climax by labour. I suspect it's a scheme sponsored by NCT to get people more into natural births, backed up by the kind of women who swear anal sex is pleasurable.

even fancy eating again if there wasn't someone squeezing my stomach to half its normal size. It would be the end of everyone touching me and talking to me. I was so sick of people laughing – actually laughing – when they saw my bump. It was a kindly 'Ho ho ho, not long now, eh?' kind of laugh, not like a maniacal one, but it was still getting really old really fast. I wasn't used to people commenting on my body. It was like I was wearing the fact that I'd been fucking right there in front of everyone, never more so than when I bumped into the vicar from my primary school, bump in full bloom.

It's suddenly OK to reach out to touch strangers and do you know what? If you're not Natalie Portman, it really isn't. Especially when your hand is a bit low and in danger of brushing the massive vagina, which might be higher than you'd expect. Just stay safe and keep your hands to yourself. And your opinions, especially when they are:

1. 'You are so massive, I hope the bag is packed and by the front door?'

2. 'WOW, you're really huge!'

3. 'You're carrying all up front – you must be having a boy.'
   'I'm having a girl.'
   'Nope, no chance. It's a boy for sure. Or a he-she.'

4. 'Do you worry that the baby will be so big you'll need one of those C-sections, where they cut you straight down the middle?'

5. 'Did you hear about that woman who died in childbirth last week? Isn't it crazy that it still happens so often in this day and age?'

6. 'Ah, my sister-in-law was a bit sick – have you tried ginger tea?'

Yes, thank you very fucking much! I have tried everything and nothing works.

So, suffice it to say, I was keen to get the baby out. Still a week from my due date I went back into hospital as my GP conceded I was massive and the PEP was a bit crazy. The gynaecologist I'd seen right from the beginning was waiting for me when without even letting her say hello or take me into a room, I begged for her to perform a C-section there and then.

'I'll paaaaaaaay!!' I insisted, though of course I wouldn't – as IF I had enough for a down payment on a C-section! I probably couldn't even get one on finance! *Damned passion-for-fashion career, why didn't I go into medicine or law? Damn you, Anna Wintour!*

'Don't be bloody ridiculous, Grace. You are a healthy young woman. Yes, you're massive, but the head's engaged and you're fine. More than capable of having this baby naturally. Bloody C-section! HA!'

I realised then I was never going to get one just by asking nicely.

I scrambled around for my birth plan when we got home. I'd glibly told the poor midwife, my only plan was NOT to vomit when she'd pressed me for one. I've always had a phobia of vomiting and so this was the main thing to avoid, in my mind. I couldn't be arsed because I knew I planned to get a C-section and clearly couldn't tell HER that! So I kept it vague. She wrote down, *Grace does not want to vomit* and we left it at that. But now I needed to get planning.

'Rich, I still think the most important bit is that I don't vomit. So … how can we action that?'

'Um, your body will just do it if it needs to. I don't know –'

'No, no, NO, I will not vomit, so what could cause that and I'll just avoid it?'

'Errrr … something with morphine in it, so pethidine? I guess?'

'GREAT! Write down: no pethidine. Say I'm allergic. What else?'

'Well, I think gas and air can make you feel a bit queasy sometimes?'

'Right, no gas and air. Hey, we're on a roll! Now, what about an epidural? Sick?'

'Nope, it blocks the pain receptors that –'

'FABULOUS! We'll have one of those, and I'll just listen to my hypnobirthing MP3. Now, how about those ice chip things? They shouldn't make me sick, if from a safe water source?'

'Yes, ice is fine … I think. Um, bubs, you might want to think about some of the stuff we talked about in NCT classes. Like the birthing pools and forceps and an episiotomy –'

'What's an episiotomy?'

'It's where they cut your va –'

'NO! Next!'

'Forceps?'

'I just don't think anything should be going *in* when we're trying to get something *out*, you know? If it really is anything like having a poo, I don't think insertion is The One. Unless it's an enema. But it doesn't seem like the time for one of those. If they offer an enema, I'll take it though. So, no to forceps, yes to an enema. Hey, and maybe the sucking thing, they could do that sucky, vacuum thing. The Vogue-douche?'

'Ventouse?'

'Yep, I'll have one of those, too. Write it down.'

Happy that my plan involved numbing and sucking, I was actually quite cheerful for the first time in weeks.

Nesting, A.K.A. watching *Real Housewives of New York* with a Twix

Firstly, I was decidedly unbothered about dirt in our house. I mocked up an attempt to clean the floor once, labouring over the corners and groaning as I couldn't see the mop beyond my massive bump, only because I thought it might guilt Rich into agreeing to sell his car and get a cleaner instead. But I was still quite anti clutter, and by that I mean The Baby Stuff. Our new home was basically a Wendy house, and we'd had to hock our sofas which wouldn't have even got through the door, instead buying a small two-seater which should have been called a one-pregnant-person-seater as it turned out. I didn't then fancy filling the remaining space with baby stuff.

I put candles around the room, hung photographic prints of naked women by Helmut Newton and Mary McCartney, trying to squeeze the twee out of the cottage and keep the Brighton edge. I was looking more and more like a country mum, so I started wearing a lot of leopard print and black in an effort to claw back my London life, the last-ditch attempt to de-mum myself. I saw Jamie Laing from *Made in Chelsea* wearing one of my tops on the show and rather than feeling disgusted with myself, I was quietly reassured.

My mum was doing my head in. She'd been this towering inferno of strength and kickass power, and now she was perpetually worried. She was either sending me articles about pre-eclampsia and skin-to-skin bonding in birth or she was tiptoeing around my black moods, with that expression that screams, 'I'm not going to say it, but …'

Where was the sassy, 'fuck'em all' woman I'd grown up with, who bemoaned the boring mums in our lives and instilled in me a sense that I could do anything? She was my role model for motherhood. Why was she being so wet about everything? And where had the sudden fascination with dribble bibs and breast pumps come from?

She wanted me to shop for the baby, clean up for the baby, start thinking about names, schools, godparents and what would the baby call her?

'Errr, Grandma?'

'God no, I'm too young! Frances's granddaughter calls her Mimi – what about that?'

'Sure, whatever, Mum, it's fine.'

'Or TT, because I'm the Timothy grandmother?'

'SURE, MUM, THAT'S FINE.'

'Or maybe GG – could be like Glam Gran …'

Rather than feeling comforted and looked after, I felt suffocated. She was in such a hurry to get me to the mum bit, while I was still hanging onto my life, losing grip fingernail by fingernail. On the flipside though, I knew she had nursed me through every ailment I'd ever had so I'd decided I definitely wanted her to be at the birth. I'd gone from thinking, *not on your life*, to thinking, *well, how can I possibly do it without her and her homeopathic goody bag of sugar pills*? There was no way I could cope without her to be the strong one. Rich was great but he was way too stoic – I needed someone who would know when to ask for the drugs, and the right lies to tell me when I shat myself.

Needless to say, Rich wasn't thrilled about this.

'I think it should just be you and me. She might get a bit stressed in that setting, she doesn't even like hospitals, for God's sake!'

'Well, darling, I understand of course, but given that it's ME who will be giving birth, I think I'll have whoever I damn well WANT in that room. OK?' Rich mumbled assent, but I think probably he thought we'd cross that bridge when we came to it.

I get it though – I wouldn't have let *his* mum in the room if she'd brought a big fat epidural with her. Plus, my mum and I were rowing fairly constantly at this point.

I felt bad for being consistently moody, and agreed to push the pram she'd forced me to buy (admittedly, from a charity shop, but still) around her garden once she'd cleaned it. Just me in my wellies, pushing an empty pram around their garden. Normal. I let her have a key to our house, and regularly came home to a bag full of babygros or toys, alongside the pathetic-looking eBay purchase of just the one second-hand Boden cardigan I'd allowed myself.

Of course, she was changing, too. She was moving from a mum to a grandmother. She was buying all the things she couldn't afford first time round, and becoming terrified by the prospect of the birth, which would potentially put her child and her grandchild at risk.

But I was hot-headed and hormonal.

NCT/Tinder for Parents

As you teeter on the precipice between your old self and the new you, you're forced to make friends via Tinder-for-parents: NCT. The NCT classes are weird, by the way. Someone gives detailed information about what your vagina will go through shortly, in front of seven other couples you've never met before. And the real agenda for probably 75 per cent of the participants is actually to pick new friends from the other 14 people (I don't include the teacher because surely nobody does that?). So, you make shit jokes, kick your husband when he says something dumb about nipple tweaking and try not to hear the stuff about tearing your perineum.

I was anxious to make new friends because I was already keenly aware that since we'd moved to the countryside and I'd left work, my friends had dropped off the radar. Before I got pregnant I had a lot of friends. In fact, I didn't believe 'best' was a superlative – they were all my best friends. You know, that kind of female friendship group fetishised by *Sex and The City*? I was in that gang! I was that cliché in stilettos, going to the loo in packs and sloshing cocktails about, sharing clothes but NEVER boyfriends. I had a very clear friend code that was far better formed than my moral outlook on the world at large. Over the years, friends made me resolutely me, they knew every secret, mishap and triumph that had shaped me.

Friends help mould and then evolve your identity, they affirm it and bolster it, and bounce it back to you in times of crisis. They call bullshit when you're kidding yourself – '*He's not worth your tears, and you never liked that cowlick in his hair, anyway*' – and give you the leg-up required when you do need to kid yourself into bravely stepping into the unknown. Anytime your identity is under fire – a cheating lover, a workplace drama, a family row, a shit fringe – you grab a friend to check you're actually unchanged, that you're still you, no matter what. What could be better fuel for our identities than to feel chosen by another person? A friend who wants to know what you think and feel about things, whether it's the Syrian refugee crisis or if socks-and-platforms is something that can actually work IRL. True friends know you when you don't know yourself. Jesus, I know – it's like I'm sat in a pink-skied tableau on Instagram, these life-affirming memes passing over my head in a curly font. You can have that one, Insta fans. But seriously, I love friends hard. I was a friend before I could read or write, before I knew who I would be, way, way before I was a wife or a mum, before I was a woman.

I'd imagined these friendships would get stronger with a baby added to the mix – friends are always there in a crisis, and in moments of joy they really come into their own, so however this whole thing went down, I knew they'd be there. I envisaged them coming to hold the baby, the conversations flowing just as they always had done, but with the added thrill of a baby to pass around and coo over. They would love the baby like I did and it would bring us all closer together. And in time, I'd be back on the dance floor with them, unchanged and as ready to party as I ever was.

It took one visit from a friend to burst that bubble. She'd had to schlep down to us because I was surprisingly large and couldn't travel far anymore. I was already altered, confined to our tiny town, a three-mile radius from our home. We met in town and a bit of wee came out as I gave up trying to control my bladder after my long walk. Finally, we ended up in a pub – I didn't want to be there, it smelt of fusty carpets and stale beer, but I didn't want to be THAT mum-to-be, so I tried to look nonchalant as she ordered a glass of wine. We spent the next couple of hours chatting about work and mutual friends and all the impending birth stuff. A man shuffled in, sat down on the table next to us and vomited into his fedora. She rolled her eyes and giggled. I wanted to go home. Soon she had to leave anyway to make the return schlep to London. We slowly ambled – waddled – back to the station to say goodbye. My baby literally came between us, kicking my friend off us as she gently pushed against me in a failed hug.

'Right, when are you next in London then?'

I paused – surely it was fairly obvious a trip to London was now unlikely? I was huge, I'd wet myself and I'd had to take my shoes off when we got to the station because my feet had doubled in size.

'Um, I don't think I will make it up again now.'

'Well, try. Because we probably won't see you once the baby's arrived.'

It hit me in the chest like a wrecking ball: I *was* going to change and nobody would want me anymore.

I was scared but also livid because it felt like I was being abandoned to this new life, like my friends didn't want to be a part of it. I mean, this particular friend and I had continued to see each other when she'd lived in another continent for a couple of years, and yet here I was having a baby and falling off the map entirely. I know, she probably didn't mean it like that, but when you're hormonal and clinging onto your old life, not yet realising how great your new life might be, you take a sentence like that at face value. And ultimately she was right – we wouldn't really see each other.

Around that time my mum asked if I'd like a baby shower. When I was bleeding and itching at intervals from the stretch marks, had no friends to speak of and was heading into what felt like another bout of antenatal depression.

'FUCK THAT', I hissed.

Instead she took me out for a cup of tea and a slice of cake at the garden centre with her friend, Marlene. They were all out of cake so I was fucking livid, but Marlene said she could read our fortune in loose-leaf tea, and when she held up the cup there was a tiny smiley face, perfectly formed amongst the brown specks.

I was really excited about NCT classes because it was our one shot at having some friends. If we had to make a change, I was ready for phase three: the friends I'd have dinner parties with and lock-ins at the local, and holidays where you fall asleep drinking red wine and playing cards, like I'd seen my parents do in their 40s. Anyway – back to NCT.

Obviously when we got the group email confirming our start time and the address, I checked out the addresses for clues. *The Body Shop – promising, I know about that stuff – and NHS, might be a doctor, that would be handy … Wait, bloody Hotmail?! Sorry, what is this – 1998?!*

We pulled up to a community centre, half nursery school, and half dodgy-looking cafe. Rich was not looking forward to this whole experience.

'I *have* friends, I don't *NEED* new ones.'

'Where are they, though, Rich?'

He mumbles unintelligibly.

'PARDON?'

'BARNSLEY!!!!'

'Right, so let's go.'

We were the first ones in, Rich dawdling at the entrance while I strode in belly-first, to meet the teacher who was setting out chairs in a circle. She was a very slight lady with a neat bob and an exceptionally friendly but gentle grin. Immediately I wondered if she might come with me when I went into labour because she seemed like she could handle it. She sensed Rich's reticence and my overbearing desperation and instructed us to sit down and write our baby's due date and sex if known, plus any nicknames or even birth names we had picked out for it. Good to keep both of us busy, Rich so he didn't leave and me so I didn't ask her to be my birth partner just yet.

Couple after couple quickly joined us. A quick scan of the room and I had clocked Ray-Bans, Mulberry bag, MAC Lady Danger lipstick. I know how this sounds, but these are the only visual markers I can identify and understand when a group of people are plastered with the same nervous smiles. Plus, I am not ageist. I assumed we would be the youngest because I had this weird conviction we were way too young to be procreating. We were actually the same age as a lot of them, but they still seemed way more grown-up.

To break the ice, our NCT guide – we'll call her Lucy – asked us to read out the baby info we'd jotted down and to introduce ourselves. I'll change their names because I don't want them to hate me. Sam, Steve and Bean; John, Emily and Pickle; Susie, Aaron and Peanut, and so on. Then began the awkward jokes which are always how I establish crushes on people. One dad

– we'll call him Scott – said, 'We've nicknamed our baby Slug, because we were in the Slug & Lettuce pub when he was conceived.' *YES! Funny! Thank fuck for that, we will probably go on holiday together and look back on this and LAUGH!*

So that exercise finished and I felt confident this was going to go well. Everyone was nervously tittering but also looked relieved that we were all nice and nobody had said anything racist yet. Then Lucy broke the mood.

'So, first of all, let's dive straight in – here are some pictures of the cervix and a baby, and I want you – as a group – to put them in the right order as labour would progress.'

'IS THAT TO SCALE?' I shrieked as I looked at the head breaking the woman's vagina open. Even as a cross-section she looked very neat one minute and then like the Dartford bloody tunnel the next.

Another teacher was brought in to tackle the question of breastfeeding.

'At first, it will seem as though there isn't much milk, but on days one, two and three, you're giving the baby colostrum, and that's so rich, they'll be full up quite quickly.'

The father in cords put up his hand.

'Yes, um, Charlie, is it?'

'Yes, hi. So, can we squeeze the breasts and sort of dribble the colostrum into the baby's mouth if they don't feed right away?'

'Um, why do you ask?'

'With cattle, if the calf won't feed right away, they sort of back the heifer into a corner of the barn and squeeze its teats into the calf's mouth. I just thought we could do the same with Jo's teats?'

I thought Charlie must be a farmer, but it turned out he was actually an accountant, so that was weird.

We all have our ways of assimilating all this rather shocking information. One woman asks many questions about sex – do nipple tweaks really speed things up? If you want to have sex, will the hospital put you in a private room? How soon after birth will we be able to have sex again? – and at some point Rich decided her husband must be hung and we solemnly named him Donkey Dick, though not to his face OBVIOUSLY. One woman interrupted Lucy many times to relate whichever topic we were on to who did the best deal on relevant materials – the cheapest breast pads, nappies, sanitary towels, nursing bras, Inca pads – I felt like she might have been sponsored. She is definitely a vlogger now. And another woman – a nurse – thankfully added her medical knowledge and work with newborns to fill in some of the gaps. And because the sole agenda of the NCT, it seems, is to persuade us all to birth as naturally as possible, this was a godsend although at the time shit me up a bit.

I made crass jokes the entire time, another woman rarely looked up from her notebook and one seemed super-casual about the whole thing, on the verge of not being bothered at all. Truth is, we were all nervous, and acting out in some way to affirm some part of us was a strength. There was a sense of extremes from the get-go. But what else do you expect from a group of women discussing the impending annihilation of their vaginas and life as they know it in front of a room full of strangers? The identity crisis is nigh, people! One woman relies on her shopping prowess, another on her medical knowledge, me on … rhyming things with vagina.*

---

* I just got schmagina. That's it.

The thing I hadn't really considered is that the NCT is very much about NATURAL Childbirth, i.e. via the vagina.

'Lucy, I will most likely have a C-section because I'm having twins, so –'

'No reason why you should need a C-section.'

'Well, I'm having twins, so –'

'Nope, you can still deliver vaginally.' I half-expected her to stick her fingers in her ears and shout LALALALA next, but we got the picture – we'd need to Google C-sections. I was still fairly convinced I'd have a C-section so I persevered.

'Lucy, I have a tilted uterus, which might make the journey out of the birth canal tricky.'

'Nonsense, all uteruses can birth perfectly naturally –'

'But Lucy, mine is very tilted. It's like the Leaning Tower of Pisa in uterine form. And it isn't elastic at all. When I had my first smear the doctor said it wasn't very elastic. Do you think I might just not be elastic enough? I mean, can you tell from the outside? What if it isn't elastic enough to stretch?'

Poor Lucy. But she was good at dispelling myths.

'I heard drinking castor oil and eating pineapple could induce labour?'

'Actually, castor oil just gives you diarrhoea, and we don't officially recommend it. But a good night of sex is actually proven to help.'

Me: 'Does it *have* to be good sex?'

Rich: 'And, like, a whole night?'

There was the odd giggle but we meant it.

When we all partook in a room-temperature cup of squash after the first hour it was clear there was already a divide forming. I'm still not sure what did it, it wasn't age related, but by the second week, five couples had started to group together, quietly comparing notes, agreeing to share tours of the hospital's labour ward. Then there were the other four – us included – who were noisy and giggling too much, interrupting Lucy's flow with our juvenile asides. I think actually it was a divide between those who were taking it seriously and those who were desperate for a social life.

Rich and I couldn't work out how to make the first move with the couples in our clique. Each night ended with, 'see you next week then!' but no social plans. Everyone was working. Rich gave me a pep talk before the fourth session.

'You need to just go for the mums, they're the keepers of the diaries. I can't crack on to those lads without sounding desperate. And I do NOT want to have to play golf. So … you do it.'

'I will, Rich. Yeh. And you know what? I'm not even nervous. You know why? Because I'm actually pretty fucking cool, me. I mean, they'd be lucky to have a friend like me, right?'

'In many ways, yes.'

'YES! LET'S DO THIS!'

Rich and I were just pulling into the car park when Lou – my favourite of the women – and her husband pulled up.

'LET THEM GO, DICKHEAD!' I hissed at Rich, waving at them and grinning.

Lou wound down her window.

'Hiya, love, you all right?'

'JUST BEEN TO HOMESENSE! BOUGHT A SOFA!' I shouted, 'AND AN OTTOMAN! WE GOT AN OTTOMAN!'

'… OK! See you in there!'

Shit, I'd been over-eager.

'That was over-eager, bubs. Try to be cool, just a bit.'

'Yes, I know that, Rich, thank you very fucking much! I'm trying. I just really like her.' I couldn't work out why I was finding it so difficult to make friends in a straightforward way, but there was no way yet of working out genuine common ground.

'Just don't try, that'll be better.'

Luckily, Lucy was on it, and after the last session we were all encouraged to go to a local pub for celebratory drinks. The womenfolk had to stay for an extra hour to discuss sanitary pads so the boys set off, looking shy and sheepish. When we joined them an hour later, it was clear they had been drinking, some more heavily than others. Rich more heavily than everyone.

'Tell me about Plum Club, Grace.' One dad sidled up just as I was politely chatting dado rails with Lou.

'Um, sorry?' I asked, knowing full well that Rich had thought it would be a brilliant icebreaker to introduce the other dads (DADS, for fuck's sake) to the concept of leaving one or both testicles hanging out of your trousers in a public setting, like an NCT class, until someone notices. I daren't look down but I gave Rich the look that said, 'I'm trying to make new friends who don't know you used to be a wine-downing bellend, please CEASE AND DESIST!' and he duly turned round and rummaged in his trousers for a moment. *I will not have him ruin this – potentially our only chance to make friends in the local area.*

A slightly scaled-back version of our group decided to go for supper, but still – FRIENDS. We ended up at our local and when we arrived, I realised two of the other dads were also drunk, while Rich appeared to have sobered up a bit, thanks to the car journey, throughout which I had threatened to leave him if he kept on drinking. It was a case of Dads Gone Wild within an hour. One jumped up on the table in the beer garden and promptly broke the table; the other kept shouting 'ZE GERMANS ARE COMING', presumably pertaining to an earlier joke. They all did Plum Club, one resting his left testicle on my shoulder while I tried to explain the ways in which Rich hadn't always been such a dick. They were all laughing as he regaled them with stories of horrific drinking injuries and his crudest jokes, and then I realised, Rich was just letting loose and making friends the only way we knew how – by getting drunk and showing off. Why should this social situation – a gathering of terrified parents-to-be – be any different?! The galling thing was, it totally worked. It might not have been very Cath Kidston behaviour, but they liked him. Meanwhile, I was sober and trying so hard to say the right things that my mouth had dried up and my upper lip was twitching. I tried to distract one of the mums away from the scene unfolding out of the window – her husband was trying to piece the broken table back together using his shoe.

'So, do you think the mucus plug is, like, solid?'

'Oh god, I couldn't give a fuck –'

'ME NEITHER! God, no, me neither – ugh, what a bore!'

I was exhausted and so relieved when the landlord basically asked us to leave. I heaved a sigh (and possibly an involuntary spot of wind) as Rich shut the car door.

'OK, Rich, you were right – we don't need new friends. I think we're fine as we are, babe.'

'WHAT? Grace, those guys are BRILLIANT! We're all going to the races next week, stick it in the diary.'

PART II

THE STRUGGLE

CHAPTER FOUR

BIRTH

I was still five days short of my due date when 16 September was just an hour away and I felt or somehow sensed a large 'POP' somewhere near my hip as I rolled over in bed. But that pop, the bursting of the sack of fluid that held my future locked up inside me, was when the old me began to die. Even in labour I was not myself – everything I did was completely out of character. And of course when I washed the debris from my legs hours later, the new me was baptised in a bath full of blood and bodily fluids. The 'new mum' was someone else entirely and not at all what anyone – least of all, what I – was expecting. Yes, the old me died that day, but the me that rose from the ashes was not at all who any of us was expecting, right from the moment labour began.

Giving birth is unlikely to affirm the ideas you had about yourself. It takes us all by surprise in one way or another, and with all the planning we're encouraged to do, it can also totally let us down, which only causes more angst and self-doubt. Birth is not just about your baby but also about the new you coming to the world. You don't know until the baby arrives exactly how you'll feel or be as a parent. Suddenly the hypothetical decisions you've made are relegated as the reality of another person's life shatters everything you thought you knew about yourself as a mum. It's all a mystery but fuck it, you're in love.

Birth plan: do not puke. Or shit

I watched a few episodes of *One Born Every Minute* when I was safely years away from even thinking of having kids. I used to laugh at it from my ivory tower of intact vaginas. It was like a really intense episode of *Big Brother*, but instead of watching people fight over food and camera time, I was watching a lot of fannies gaping around massive baby heads. I got into a predictable cycle with each episode – I'd start off stoic, then get a little grossed out and cover my eyes at the rank baseness of it all. I'd most likely sneer at the inept husbands – *haha, what a prick!* – or the banter between midwives, but then I'd always start screaming as heads crowned and things spurted out, and then without fail, I'd cry. Every time a baby was hoisted up in the air, I was sobbing. Weird, because I pretty much hated babies and kids, but maybe it was a biological thing I still can't grasp. With the exception of a girl who birthed almost silently in a pool (*I'll probably do it like that*, I Tweeted at the time), the women I saw were wild, untidy and gurning, overcome by what seemed like a brutish, violent process. I just couldn't imagine ever letting myself go feral like that because I'd never experienced that pain or urge to make like a defecating panda in front of other people. My mum warned me off watching it as 'they only pick the dramatic ones and you don't need that'. This from the woman who told me every detail of the birth – *my* birth – that nearly killed her and left her paralysed for 10 days. So once I was pregnant I swore off all programmes related to pregnancy or birth (apart from *16 and Pregnant*, which was strangely comforting – if these children can do it, maybe I can handle it after all).

By the time my baby was fully gestated and that popping sensation occurred, I was a safe distance from all memories of seeing a crowning head or a woman mooing in a hot-tub filled with what I'd assumed was red wine. But, I was also well conditioned to think I was a wimp. I was pretty sure I'd be a car crash unless they performed a C-section, so I just decided that's how I'd roll. Plus, I was so bloody sick of being pregnant, I wanted it all over with. It was a mixed bag of emotions.

Now you wouldn't be blamed for thinking, shit this is going to be bad. This woman can't handle labour! It's a really bloody and painful thing, she sounds a bit neurotic so she's just going to panic or bribe someone to give her a C-section. That was my plan actually, which is possibly why I felt so relaxed. If I could just rest for a bit, someone would eventually step in and take over – a professional – and I would just do as I was told, with oodles of pain relief. Once the vomiting started, I'd ask for help, OK? Cool. I didn't feel nauseous, which had always been my main concern, so I just fixed on getting to the point where a midwife wouldn't send me home and I'd be welcomed in to be rubbed and injected until the baby was born. When I was about four I was obsessed with giving birth – I'd receive an injection and then pull a doll out from under my T-shirt. My cousin almost ruined it for me by saying babies actually come out of the fanny, but my mum's crude description of an epidural sufficed and I'd still go for the injection followed by a dignified removal of doll from knickers. I'd clearly carried this game with me into adulthood and even now I was all about the injection that would save me the blood, sweat and tears. I didn't believe in heroics – I would not go through hell with the same result in mind just so I could say I'd done it.

Just as I started to tell Rich about the weird popping sensation, a great flash flood gushed through my pants, soaking our bed sheets. Having heard it's nothing like the movies when your waters break, that there's rarely a big gush of fluid, it was *exactly* as I'd imagined it. It didn't hurt so I was more amused than anything, especially as Rich seemed to be having a breakdown mid-flow.

'Oh fuck, oh fuck, it's happening. OK, OK. Stop! Now, stop it! It's going EVERYWHERE!' My usually insanely relaxed husband was flapping. He was throwing towels at me, trying to wedge one under me. It was really funny.

I was hysterical.

'Now that's what I call a baby shower – it's like ejaculating all over the bed, hahaha!'

'No, don't laugh! It's gushing, it's fucking gushing, STOP!'

'OK, get me to the loo, it's the only way,' I eventually choked out, laughing again as he pulled me to my feet and immediately wedged the already soggy towel between my thighs. I dripped a trail to the bathroom, and the water continued to leak out into the loo, eventually slowing to a trickle and finally a drip-drip … drip. Rich was carefully studying my face, I could tell. Then he started shining a torch between my legs into the toilet bowl.

'Dude, what the fuck?!'

'I'm checking the waters, to see if they're clear. They need to be clear, don't they? If they're brown it means the baby's pooed inside you.'

'Sorry, *WHAT*?!'

I realised then and there I really hadn't paid any attention in our NCT classes. I was busy thinking about who we'd most likely go on holiday with when all this was done, if the shoes I was wearing projected the right kind of vibe ('capable but quite fun and obviously, impossibly glamorous' – a lot to pin on a pair of patent leather brogues). I hadn't read the birth chapters in *What To Expect When You're Expecting*. In fact, the only things I could remember from any literature was that Cathy had died giving birth in *Wuthering Heights*, and that Caitlin Moran's second birth had been better because she'd kept moving. But now Rich – who it seemed had gleaned bits of information concerning this present predicament – seemed stressed. I tried to comfort him.

'I'm fine, relax, bubs! I think although that flash flood was a bit OTT, it'll still be like a week or something before I go into labour.'

Rich began to Google things, and wandered off upstairs to check out the leaflets stuffed in the Purple Folder. He came back down swallowing nervously, his pace slower, his eyes wide.

'You have 24 hours from now.'

I was weirdly relaxed. Like, not worried a jot, not even full of butterflies or buzzing. I had listened to a hypnobirthing MP3 when I was about five months pregnant, so maybe it had seated itself somewhere in my brain? God knows where my iPod was that night though, and is the one listen really enough to master the art of visualising a baby out of you? Or maybe that plastic syringe from my childhood doctor's kit was acting as a cerebral comforter as my cervix got to stretching.

I got back into bed, pants stuffed with pads the size of bricks, and must have slept for a couple of hours because suddenly it was 1am. I had some gentle period pains so got up to move about a bit, pop a couple of paracetamol and find the birthing ball.

'Is it happening?' Rich murmured, sitting bolt upright but with his eyes shut.

'No, bubs, go back to sleep. It'll be hours yet.'

I sat in our cool, dark living room. There were no streetlights in our little village and there wasn't a single sound coming from inside or out. I considered what was happening – the baby is coming; this is it for sure now. But still I didn't feel anything close to what such a momentous thing should surely trigger. I didn't feel emotional. In fact, I've cried more during especially threatening bowel movements. I moved around our little house, bouncing around on a yoga ball, floating from one contraction to the next like those women I read about but never believed in.

Time just passed without me noticing. I didn't clockwatch (we didn't have a clock yet) so I was surprised when Rich came down to tell me it was 5.30am.

'I think we should go into the hospital now,' he murmured quietly, like Clive Mantle in *Casualty*, he'd obviously been perfecting his bedside manner while upstairs.

'Bubs, I'm fine, honestly.' I was aware I was biting my lip gently so tried to smile to convey utter calm.

'Yeh. OK. Well, how far apart are the contractions?'

'Um, like … maybe every three minutes?' I guessed because frankly, who the hell knew?

'Three?! OHMYGOD, WE HAVE TO GO, WE HAVE TO GO NOW'

'Oh no, not three then. Maybe … 10 minutes?'

This didn't seem to placate Rich, who was now keen to hand over control to the midwives rather than deliver the baby himself. He made me speak to a midwife so she could gauge how close I was to needing assistance and settle the impending row between us.

'You sound OK, sweetheart, *are* you OK?' She sounded kind and tired, and ever the people pleaser, I agreed – I really was fine.

'OK, well, call the community midwife when she starts her shift at 8am and she'll pop in to see you on her rounds. Her number's in your notes. And maybe have a bath if the pain gets stronger before that.'

She rang off and I smugly returned to the living room and took up my post on the ball, gracefully face-planting the sofa. Rich scurried upstairs to Google 'home delivery'.

After a while, I went back upstairs, meaning to find the Jelly Babies I'd packed in my hospital bag. Rich was sat up in bed.

'OK, I think it's time to go now, bubs. Let's just go in, get checked out. You look kind of warm, are you hot? It says here if you get a temperature we should go into the hospital.'

I was too busy chewing on the throw at the end of the bed to respond, but I let him put a cool hand to my forehead.

I got the sense he was a little agitated. But I just couldn't be arsed, you know? It seemed like a right bloody mission, getting stuff in the car, driving, sitting and stuff. I was just not in enough pain yet to be interfered with and I felt pretty fucking Zen here at home. It would clearly still be hours and hours until anything really happened, so why haul ass to the hospital when I was just fine at home? I was so convinced I would feel abject pain before most people did that I'd be 1cm dilated for a week or so and I thought to myself, until it's making me want to vomit, I'll just sit it out. Years of IBS spasms had prepared me for this. How different could this be, really, except that I hadn't eaten any Chinese food to trigger it?

I was so sure midwives would be spending days telling me I was nowhere near. That's how my birth experience would be – professionals telling me I was wrong and my instincts were off and I needed to wait longer.

'Yeh, you're hot, I think you're hot. I'm going to call them again.'

'I'm totally fine,' I mumbled as another wave crested and I gripped the bed.

'Hi, it's me again. She's really hot … yes. Right, yes, OK. We'll come now.'

I was so not hot but he couldn't handle it anymore.

Rich began rushing up and down to pick up a bag, then another, then another, trying to chivvy me along while I waddled along, stopping every couple of steps for a little sit down. He ran from the car to me, the car and back to me again, and in a moment free from his rushing I looked around our living room for a split second, saying goodbye to life as we knew it.

It would look the same when we got back, I knew, but what would *we* look like? When would we be coming back? The house still felt so new, but already it was my me-shaped sanctuary, with my books and my cushions and the print I'd found wedged behind my desk at *Vogue* and had carried from flat to flat. How would this all work with another person taking up a spot on the sofa, where would all my stuff *go* when this new person arrived? I wasn't scared exactly, just aware this was one of those big moments and I was just a naïve, inexperienced version of who I was about to become. It was the last time I looked around at my life for a second without feeling guilty for being selfish and self-involved. Those questions I had were all about me, how I would reconcile the changes, and I felt no shame in that.

Then I actually thought for a moment, *what if I don't come back? What if it's Rich coming back alone, or with a baby, but without me?* But just as the thought crossed my mind, another surge came and I closed my eyes, riding my ball like a space hopper, down the path to the car.

The car ride was surprisingly OK – everything stopped for a while. The speed bumps at the hospital were NOT OK. Who puts speed bumps that close to a maternity ward? I'm pretty sure those alone caused an extra few centimetres of cervix to just crank right open. Rich stopped the car in front of the entrance and ran to the intercom since it was only 6am and pretty dark outside. I wasn't really aware of what was happening by now, the contractions were making me feel a bit absent from the real world. But he had to run from the intercom, get buzzed in and then run back to me, trying to coax me to walk the two metres to the door before it locked again. I feel like the *Benny Hill* theme tune must have been playing throughout. He did this about seven times – I was always waiting for a contraction to end – and then finally he yanked on my arms to winch me out.

'Come ON, ferfucksake, Grace, get OUT!'

Walking wasn't great but I managed a good pace considering my vagina was dropping down to my knees. I did little circuits of the lift, rubbed my thighs and DING we arrived. The assessment unit was empty. We were directed by a receptionist to a room with three curtained beds, where someone would come and take us through the paperwork when they were free.

Things felt a bit more urgent now.

'Shit, Rich! Shit! This is getting a bit tricky now. Woooooooooo!'

'Grace, just please try not to swear so much, the receptionist is the mum of a guy I work with. I don't want –'

'FUCK OFF, YOU FUCKING TWAT!'

'Fine. OK, fine.'

I paced round the room, climbed on and off the bed, bounced on the ball. Everything inside me seemed to be gathering now – there seemed to be a lot of things poised to drop out, heavy things, possibly bricks, dragging everything else south. I hung off Rich's collar (kudos to River Island, it didn't rip …), trying to ground myself but stay upright. Having sworn I wouldn't do it, I started mooing and bossed Rich out into the hallway to find a midwife.

'Don't come back until you have one of those bitches with you, all right?'

Rich couldn't find anyone and came back with a receptionist, who asked me to wee in a pot in her bored voice. Rich and I hobbled to the loo and I peeled the massive sanitary towel out of my pants.

'Hold this – they need to see this. Hold it for the midwife.'

'What?! No! I don't want to hold … THAT! Why do they need to see it?'

'They've got to check the blood or the wee or something – OH CHRIST, HERE COMES ANOTHER ONE!'

Then suddenly it was like my labour started in earnest – the pain kicked in, I felt this innate shudder course through my body, which felt like the urge to vomit but in reverse, so that rather than everything shooting up from stomach to throat, it was like everything was careering down to my knees. Sitting down and weeing seemed entirely out of the question and blood started to trickle out into the bowl Rich was trying to hold beneath me. A midwife heard me shouting, 'I can't wee, I can't WEEEEEEE!' and helped Rich guide me back to the examination room. I was making *that* noise, the noise that alerted those in the know to a large dilation of the cervix. I writhed around on the bed, now feeling pain pulsing around my cervix, up and down my legs, all across my lower belly, and she checked me over.

To everyone's surprise I was 10cm dilated, my baby's head was crowning and it was time to push.

Errrrr, what? I hadn't got in a pool, or had a foot massage, or listened to my playlist, had an epidural, or even eaten a single Jelly Baby! I hadn't spritzed my face with spring water! I hadn't even got changed beyond whipping my knickers off. I wasn't ready! Rich stepped in, taking his role as 'advocate' very seriously. 'Grace would like a water birth,' he told the midwife. 'Could we please move to the birthing centre, to a room with a pool?'

She replied that she'd start running a bath for afterwards if he liked but there wasn't time to get to the birthing suite. She basically told us in midwife terms, 'Not gonna happen, mate.'

The best we'd manage now was getting into a delivery room.

I bellowed 'I'm not fucking moving!' and so the midwife wheeled a cot and other equipment into the exam room while outpatients started milling about in the corridor, waiting for their check-ups. She sneezed and I pulled Rich to my face,

'If she's got a fucking cold, get her OUT OF HERE!!'

I started pushing – stopping only to fling my very expensive T-shirt, which I had NOT planned to give birth in, across the room. At 8am the midwife's shift ended but I held onto her for dear life and despite it being her wedding anniversary, she agreed to stay, working alongside her replacement. Then the baby's heart rate dropped and my energy levels with it.

'Do whatever, get it out, get it out!' I yelled incoherently, feeling my voice slipping away from me, but desperate to end this immediately.

'Get Miss Tatley!' I suddenly remembered my gynaecologist had written her mobile number in my notes with strict instructions to call her if she was needed.

'We're not going to bother her on a Sunday morning! You'll be fine,' clucked the midwife with the long hair. I wanted to pull it out of her head and strangle her with it.

The room filled with people and a young woman told us she was going to perform an episiotomy and then suck the baby's head out with a ventouse. Now, on a normal day the news that someone was poised to chop through my vagina with a pair of scissors would have made me leg it out of there, but I was so up for it I was practically leaning into her face to get it done quicker. Rich spoke up again, though. I heard a tremor in his voice.

'Grace doesn't want an episiotomy, she was very clear on that.'

I'm not sure how the registrar responded to this but I felt a splash of something thrillingly cold on my hot, throbbing vagina, which at the time I assumed was a numbing solution (haha, as if!) but was actually clearing away some of the blood so she could see what she was doing as she spliced the flesh. And there was the cut, a sharp stabbing sensation.

'FUUUUUCKIIIIIIIIIIIIING HEEEEEEEEEELL!' I screamed. But then the pain was gone as quickly as it came. It was almost a relief that the insane stretching was over, and it just felt like insane pressure. Then they sucked, I pushed and out came the head. 'STOP!' they yelled at me, and then moments later, the body slithered out at 8.25am.

Suddenly, there she was. She was swung across the bed onto my chest, my arm quickly bending around her warm little body, wrapped in a towel with a hand-knitted pink hat snapped around her rather large head. She was scrunched up and her mouth was red and wet. I looked at Rich, dumbstruck and smiling down at her. This baby had been growing inside me, had been sharing my blood and oxygen and food and heartbeat. But she wasn't an organ or a new limb, she was a person.

Because I'd not actually seen her coming out – when the registrar offered to show me her head hanging out of my vagina, I'd declined, that's fucking disturbing, but thanks – I still couldn't equate her with what had been inside my body, with the kicks and dome of a belly. I didn't feel the connection I'd expected, that kind of 'Oh, you came out of me, you were just in there and now you're out here' feeling. But I did feel I had this huge pull towards her. I don't think I felt like her mother, exactly – who would know how that was meant to feel? – but I did want to be with her all the time, forever. Rich kissed me on the head and reached down to stroke the tiny hand flailing around beneath my chin.

Hi kid, is that you? Did you really just grow inside me? Are you really all mine? She was so little compared to objects around us but so big when I considered where she'd just come from. She was blinking her big black eyes and although I knew that technically she couldn't focus yet, I was aware that my face was the first thing she'd seen on the outside. She was beginning her life, this moment was the start of it all. Eventually she would be out there in it all. I felt in that instant that she was already on her way. I couldn't believe I got to keep her. It was like having a brilliant new toy – the feeling you get when you go downstairs on your birthday or at Christmas and are given the toy you've been thinking about ever since you saw it advertised on TV. That, times a billion. I just wanted to touch her and hold her. I wanted her to open her eyes so I could make her laugh (they do that, right? Newborns laugh?), buy her all the toys in the world, and show her our home and her dad. *NOW I get it*, I thought, *having a baby really IS the best thing in the world. I couldn't care less about anything else now she's here.*

Apparently I delivered the placenta while I sat and stared at my new baby (MY baby!), and the registrar started stitching me back up but I don't remember it. She offered me gas and air for the stitches but I didn't see the point when I'D JUST PUSHED A BABY OUT WITHOUT BEING OFFERED ANY so I just fixed my eyes on the suckling baby, jerked around a little bit, and within minutes the registrar was done. And that was that. 'The next one will FLY out,' said the midwife as she rifled through the four bags we'd stacked up on the bed next door for baby clothes and nappies.

Since panic exacerbates pain and I'm an exceptionally panicky person normally, I should have been a mess. But I was left wondering whether IBS really had prepared me to withstand intense pain? Or my conviction that I was often wrong and always a wimp meant that I didn't give any weight to my own pain, didn't think I was experiencing *enough* pain for it to be active labour? I was so used to being told off for overreacting in life as a longtime drama queen, I figured I was destined to be treated with nothing short of contempt by midwives for 'wasting their time' and getting to the hospital too early, so I was prepared for a long wait until things became unbearable. I wasn't making conscious decisions throughout the labour, I was just waiting for it to kick in. And I understand how lucky I am because I know women with far less selfish outlooks and far more sensible characters who have really struggled and for whom it's been an ordeal. Maybe my slightly tilted uterus was in some way a help in the end.

Getting one's tits out

Towards the very end of my pregnancy, I remember clearly thinking, *I can't wait to get my body back*. Not get into shape and lose weight, but to get ownership and control over my body again. It was a week or two before the baby was due and I was swollen, fit to burst. I was trying to roll myself onto my side because you can't sleep on your back OR your front, of course. My skin had gone shiny, and my belly was square, as a hand jerked inside me and the curve became an angle.

As I lay there, sneaking a cheeky scratch by lying on my hand, I thought about this belly. I felt fully taken over. And when the baby was out, my body would be my own again. The hormones would finally chill, surely, and I would be back to normal, back to my old self. I was so excited.

And true enough, as soon as she was out, I felt it: I felt different. Looking at her dark eyes, her wrinkled skin and her matted hair, it was *her* – not this terrible ordeal or a nameless illness, it was all for this creature. She was out. It was over. She was lying in the crook of my right arm, a towel over us both, and I could finally feel her; her skin wasn't my skin, her limbs weren't part of my body anymore. I felt our separateness. This separateness lasted a full minute, before the midwife suggested I try breastfeeding.

'Just stick her on, see how it feels,' she said.

I awkwardly edged her up towards my chest, looking at her and my nipple, the gap between them. With the midwife's help I managed to put the whole thing in her tiny mouth, and straight away she began to suck. And with the vacuum of her mouth we were attached again. My tits became the new umbilical cord. But this time I fucking loved it. She suckled hard and I could feel the wash of calm creeping over my entire body. It was like a high I'd never experienced. So in terms of getting my body back? No, that was a really naïve idea. We'd actually be linked like this for the next THREE YEARS (yep, that long), but at this point, as a shell-shocked new mother with no expectations of anything except probable failure, it was all OK.

'I'd better go and … call someone?' Rich looked completely traumatised and wrung out now the room had cleared of people and it was just <u>us again</u>. 'I need to tell the team I won't be coming into work today, and there's our parents …'

'FUCK! I didn't call my mum!' I knew she'd be gutted to have missed it all. It hadn't even crossed my mind – I didn't feel that primal need for her to manage the situation like I'd expected.

That feels quite nice, I thought to myself, *I managed*. It had happened so quickly, and my parents were probably still asleep. Rich went out into the hallway to ring his boss first (yep), and then both sets of grandparents while I ate toast with one hand.

The midwife told me after a quick wash I could go straight home, but I asked to stay for a bit – I was worried it had all been a bit too straightforward and wanted at least a few hours in hospital in case anything ruptured or fell out of me. I was a bit concerned about the easy-breezy way they said, 'We're *pretty* sure you'll be fine'. Like, it's definitely *possible* that you'll haemorrhage and die, but hopefully not. I also wanted someone to have a good look at my asshole, because I was fairly sure I'd pushed so hard it was now on the outside of my body.

Rich had well and truly had his fill of being the responsible adult so while he left to buy supplies and just process the past eight hours, I thought I'd just find out about breastfeeding, stockpile these handy Inca pads they kept slipping into my various bags and just like, eat some more toast? I mean, I didn't know when to feed her, how often – nothing. So while I waited to see if she knew more than me, I thought it best to have some adults around me.

I practically skipped to the bathroom with the midwife, while Rich sat down with the baby in his arms for the first time. The midwife warned me against a bath – 'It'll be a total mess,' she explained – but I wanted to lie down and just look at myself for a minute. She was right though – as cathartic as it had sounded in my head to just soak the blood away and take stock, it was actually horrible, lying in a pool of my own blood and … bits of something or other. The shower was amazing – I watched the trauma circle the plughole and disappear, and took stock of my body. The bump was still there, a sort of squishy blancmange with something hard in there somewhere, but most definitely smaller and very empty. I felt lighter in every sense. Not quite as back to normal as I'd assumed – I genuinely didn't know you left hospital with a bump and had packed a pair of jeans in my hospital bag, as if I'd just jump straight back into a rigid waistband, like, SNAP, I'M BACK, BITCHEZ! But it didn't bother me because I was alive and itching to get back to the baby and Rich.

Quite a good mum, actually

So I sat in this tiny room all alone with my baby, a mere two hours after arriving in hospital, shell-shocked but grinning like an idiot. *Well, that was weird,* I thought. I knew I was really lucky that my daughter's birth went far better than I could have hoped and that I felt pretty high from the experience. Everything I did that night was completely out of character though, and again made me wonder who and what I had become. It was a brief break from the worrying about myself – I was finally solo again, nobody was living inside me, but I wasn't having to face what would happen next as we slumbered in the baby bubble, free from the outside world. She wasn't crying and so I started to wonder, am I actually quite a good mum after all?

Bless that new-mum version of me. I mean, I hadn't been faced with a single decision regarding her wellbeing, or even a single nappy for God's sake, but I was surfing the massive high of surviving the birth, and I had illusions of grandeur. I wanted to touch her and cuddle her and just give her the best life. It all felt very nice. *Wait, am I … am I an Earth Mother now?!* Shit, I could almost feel the hippyness creeping up on me. I'd just given birth with no pain relief, which yes, wasn't a conscious decision but still, I knew I'd be welcomed into those yurts full of massive-nippled women dressed in cheesecloth and linen on that basis alone.

A midwife came in to check on me, running through a checklist of questions about my labour, but I was focused on my own mental checklist as I realised how quickly I was changing already.

Do I want to just pop out and get a massage, or maybe a nice relaxing pedicure? *Nope.* What about a big night out to celebrate with all my girlfriends? *Nope.* Do I fancy a glass of wine? A cheeky little cocktail? *Nope.* Would I like to pop to TK Maxx, where they have a huge sale on and everything's basically free for a massive shopping spree? *God, no.* What about a quick, all-expenses-paid trip to New York, you love New York? *No, I'd rather stay here with her – JESUS! What have I become?*

It was nice though. Rather than fearing every second which lay ahead of me I was excited and relaxed all at once.

My mum and dad arrived soon after Rich had left, and I basked in their pride.

'Dad, I had stitches and everything, you know, in my labia and stuff, but I'm fine now!'

While Mum cradled her new granddaughter, silently weeping with joy, my dad moved on fairly quickly from my story of guts and glory.

'So, last night on stage, I was just coming up to that big monologue in act two when ...'

'No, Dad, no! But I just ... I just had a baby – like two hours ago! Isn't that amazing?'

'Amazing, darling! So there I am, about to deliver when I see a cockroach run across the stage! Can you imagine?! I mean, I got through it – it was HARD, but I got through it.'

I was taking it all in my stride, that's what it all felt like. It had all fallen into place. I was still eating, drinking, and eventually weeing. I showered, dressed, felt wildly myself again – there was no baby thrashing around, no nausea, just me. I looked down and waggled my toes – they looked the same. I looked at my sleeping baby.

When Rich came back to us I had to admit, it was turning out to be pretty easy.

'She's slept the entire time – she's just really Zen, I think. And … I think I'm a bit of an Earth Mother, you know?'

Rich definitely raised his eyebrows at this, but clearly this day wasn't one for his acerbic put-downs – BROKEN TWOT, PEOPLE! – so he nodded and handed me a bagel.

If I'd left as the kindly midwife had suggested, I'd have been home, tucked up in my own bed. The only problem is, once you're on the maternity ward you're in the system and there are certain tasks you have to perform to get released, like in *The Crystal Maze*. If you fail to produce either breast milk or urine, you'll be locked in overnight. As soon as they'd put a condition on my release I wanted it so bad. Things got markedly worse when my mum – who hates hospitals – began to recount the tale of our elderly neighbour, George, who had gone in for a routine prostate op and had never come out, pointing out the dust in the room, and someone coughing in the next room.

'You want to get this baby out of here, Grace. This place is probably CRAWLING WITH DISEASE!'

And when after two litre bottles of water I did produce urine, I knew I had to tell them right away. But I'd passed a LOT and the kidney bowl was sort of sloshing it about. I wasn't sure about carrying it back to my bed unaided. Luckily there was a handy sign next to me, instructing me to pull the red cord for assistance. Ah, like that button on planes to summon an air steward? So I pulled it. Well, all hell broke loose. An alarm went off and as I opened the door to the loo people ran at me from all directions.

'I'VE DONE A WEE!' I announced triumphantly when three nurses skidded to a stop in front of me.

They were not amused and one had to sit down because she thought she was going to sick up the tomato soup she'd been in the middle of eating. But I'd done my wee, and they promised someone would be along to sign me out as soon as possible.

And after an hour trying to fit the car seat into the car, we took our baby home.

CHAPTER FIVE

0–3 MONTHS

Broken, bleeding vagina. Thirty-six hours with no sleep. Twelve hours ago A WOMAN SCISSORED MY LABIA, AND NOT IN A SEXY WAY. And yet, I am incredibly happy. I am daft with it, giddy. I am so happy I could puke! Interesting …

Earth Mother

That night I sat in the chair we'd put in her nursery and stared at her some more. I couldn't put her down.

One of Rich's friends called and demanded to speak to me to know I definitely did survive the process.

'Yeh, and I didn't even have any pain relief,' I slurred happily, realising this is some kind of accomplishment, if you can count shitting a person out of your fanny as an accomplishment. Which I do.

Rich went to bed at around 11pm but I was far too excited to sleep. I loved the quiet as the sun slowly rose through the window, lighting up her face. So I sat there, a blanket over both of us. I uncovered her feet to see her miraculous toes, covered them again, and then snuck another look. I was sat on a pile of four sanitary pads, which felt like bricks, but as long as I didn't move I wasn't even really in any pain anymore. I caressed her forehead, her perfectly smooth, soft skin. Her puckered, swollen eyes had already calmed to perfect little mounds of featherlight skin.

I expected to come home from the hospital and immediately get back to the old me, guzzling the wine Rich had stocked the fridge with, and a ton of blue cheese, paté and cured meats. Texting mates, watching the next episode of *Dexter*, rocking the Moses basket with a foot but otherwise free to be me again. But I felt different. My old comforts still didn't appeal – I didn't need or want them. Suddenly, all that mattered was the happiness of this tiny creature that I loved so intensely even though she hadn't yet said a single word. I didn't know a single thing about her! I knew nothing, and yet I loved her without a single reservation.

I didn't even care how my new plan – to stay with her every minute of every day from now on – might impact on my career, my relationships and my ambitions – *who cares?! This is better than I've ever felt about anything, ever!* I became fully immersed in this miraculous new relationship. *I won't ever leave her, not for a second. I won't ever need a break from this. I will do everything for her.* This was very unexpected. I fully thought I'd be quite keen to make use of the new separateness and stretch my feet a bit, be on my own. But this was where I wanted to be, this was the person I wanted to be. I didn't want to be the person I had been just a few hours before. I was – and still am – head over heels with this person I didn't even know I needed. *God, if I'd met this new me the year before, I'd have hated her.*

When Rich got up that first morning and found us sitting, serene and peaceful, where he left us last night, he cocked his head to one side.

'You OK, bubs? Have you been up all night?'

'I'm fine, it's no bother.' I spoke in a low, even tone so as not to disturb the baby, but also because it sounded kind of spiritual and very much of the Madonna and Child genre I seemed to be slipping into. I thought about getting some white broderie anglaise nightgowns so I could be very bohemian and motherly all at once.

I decided to keep the fact I was forever changed a secret. Rich would definitely take the piss and I felt like I might be all out of witty retorts, grinning like an idiot. Instead I went along with our original plan to Not Change At All. It was pretty easy as it turned out.

We had to take the baby back to the hospital for the standard check-up with the paediatrician, so then we took her into town and did normal shopping and normal sandwich eating, as if everything was just as it was but we had this handy apparatus on which to put our bags. It was just really easy. She was STILL asleep, and we managed to march the length of town without her stirring. Once we'd established she was not dead, we relished the surprising ease of it all. *Maybe we really would be able to live the same lives, but it'll just feel 10 times better than before?* I was optimistic and full of love. *I really COULD have it all! There's time to work, shop, chat, eat sandwiches – but it's all better because she's here!* What could go wrong?

'I think I could actually kill someone,' I mused to Rich one afternoon. 'Maybe I'm less of an Earth Mother, more "aggressive, territorial mum" instead? Like if someone said she was not a good singer or was annoying, I think I could kill them. That's weird, isn't it?'

'Maybe don't tell the health visitor.'

Do you want to see my vagina?

The next day was a bit bleak. I didn't get the rush of tears and sadness I'd been warned to expect, but all the walking we did the day before had resulted in intense pain in the vag. It felt like I'd been punched by a truck. The new me was definitely still happier, relieved and chipper but couldn't walk without her fanny hurting.

'Rich, please, PLEASE look at my fanny! I need to know it's not infected.'

'Phrrrrrrr, no! No, I can't do that, bubs, sorry. Not ready to see … that … again.'

'Please! If it's infected I need to know!'

'Hmm. Tempting. But no.'

By the time evening rolled round, it was even tougher as the vagina-shaped ice packs weren't cutting it anymore and I knew sleep was what I needed to heal but I couldn't do it. If I moved my fanny screamed, but if I lay still it throbbed as gravity seemed to be working against me and pushing all the blood there. Rich was sympathetic, aside from the full-body shudders he did every time anyone said the word 'vagina'. He suggested he had the Moses basket on his side so he could hand the baby across to me and settle her after each feed but I didn't fancy moving her, I wanted her next to me right there. I felt safe knowing she was within reaching distance and that I could hear every snuffle. The Earth Mother stuff was getting a bit territorial now, a bit heavy, but I was still high from the mix of oxytocin and adrenalin, so it was no hardship to stay up with her. I also really wanted to do all the stuff and protect Rich from the sleeplessness.

In the morning, a midwife visited us and weighed the baby. She brought a trainee and I asked them to look at my vagina, assuming that's what they're there for.

'Well, no, not really, but … Yep, OK, then do you want to go upstairs?'

I'd already pulled down my pants and popped one leg up on the armchair.

'Oh, there you are. OK, Gemma, why don't you take this one then?'

The young trainee edged forward gingerly, snapping on a pair of latex gloves. Her nose was scrunched up as she poised a finger between my legs, and she grimaced.

'It's just bruised, love. It's … ooo, that looks painful though, doesn't it, Sue? That bit there looks … painful.'

Sue agreed.

'Is it worse than other vaginas you've seen, though, is it normal?' I asked.

Gemma looked to Sue for reassurance.

'Yes, love. I mean, no, it's all normal. Keep it clean, have a bath, get some ice on it. Right, we'll be off then!'

In the morning I was peachy actually, but for the dull ache in my pants. I hadn't done enough of the lying around, but the in-laws were due to arrive so I had to pull it together. I wanted them to see how brilliantly relaxed and unchanged we were. *You thought I'd be batshit crazy, didn't you? Well, HA! Because I am very into it and actually very good at it, fuck you very much.* Rich was grinning so hard his face might have cracked, as he pointed out the baby's button nose to his mum, and the way she pouted when she was ready to feed.

I hobbled around as they passed the baby from one to the other, squealing as my vagina made contact with a chair, electing to stand instead. I didn't feel the rush of love seeing family coo over her though, I kind of wanted them out so I could ice, bathe and then air my fanny, baby tucked in one arm. I did not enjoy knickers anymore, even the really massive ones my mum bought me from M&S. Although I was thrilled to report to my brother-in-law's new 25-year-old girlfriend that they were too big, despite the fact this was the first conversation we'd ever had.

'I think I'm probably back in my normal knickers tomorrow, actually,' I told her, snapping the elastic that sat just under my armpit.

When the family finally left I immediately took off my clothes and sobbed quietly, lying on a stack of Inca pads in our bedroom. I agreed to lie in bed for the next two days. I bathed in between feeds. Rich was endlessly patient, methodically collecting and returning the baby to me, nipping out at all hours for paracetamol, making me tea and paté sandwiches while I fed. Midwives visited every other day and I invited each one up to check out my vagina. But they didn't seem that into it. I had to really petition for that check-up. I got my mum to check, too, just for a balance of opinion. But another couple of days of baths, ice packs and a few paracetamol and it finally stopped hurting and bleeding, and we got back to getting back. We went out for supper, we visited friends, we tested out what it's like to live our pre-baby lives with a baby in tow.

One night we met up with Lou and her husband, Todd, from NCT, at our local pub for supper. It felt fairly like life before the baby, as she sat nestled in her car seat at the head of the table.

'I think I was racing Todd, you know?' Rich tells me afterwards. 'We were changing the kids and I kept trying to speed up so he'd think I was a good dad. The thing is, he put the frills of the nappy OUTside. Isn't that crazy?!'

I laughed, both at their idiocy and our supreme parenting skills.

'But we ALL know frills go on the INSIDE of the nappy, so the stuff doesn't just leak out!' We both laughed. It felt good to be right.

'HUH.' Rich was looking at his phone, reading something that made his brows knit together like snogging caterpillars. 'It says here, frills go on the outside.'

'WHAT? But that makes no sense. Clearly, if they're in, they hold in all the gumph?'

'Yeh, that said though, she has basically leaked through every nappy we've ever put her in, hasn't she?'

I consider this.

'So, Todd was right then?'

'Appears so. Shit, I wonder if he noticed me putting the frills in?'

The next day a new kind of health visitor came to the house. Not your check-out-my-vagina type or one we'd check in with regarding nappy frills, but the social worker kind who was assigned to see if you were on the verge of a breakdown yet. Or so we'd been warned by everyone we knew who had been through it. We needed to appear exceptionally happy and very responsible. After the initial pleasantries, Gill the health visitor got straight down to business.

'So, do you think you agree on what kind of parents you should be?' She poised her pencil over the form, looking up at us with no hint of a smile. *Does it actually say that on the form?!*

'Ummmmmm,' I looked to Rich for a definitive 'YES'. But he looked like he was struggling to work out the best, most believable answer to this, and which would get us on to level two of this weird parenting game with the dour-looking health visitor/game lord.

'Good … parents?' I asked, hopefully.

'Yes, well, obviously, but do you agree on the way you'll be raising this baby?'

What in the sweet hell are you supposed to say? I mean, 'yes' is obviously the one they're looking for, isn't it? But isn't it a bit insincere to say you'll always agree on everything? And ridiculous? I was also wary of seeming TOO fine, too compliant, in case they thought I was lying. Say 'NO' though and you're facing a lot of explanations as to how you'll overcome this basis of disagreement. So far we'd argued about the car seat (him: we'll just use my sister's old car seat, it's fine/me: why would you want our baby to die in a car crash?), the baby bath (him: we'll just use my sister's old baby bath, it's fine/me: why would you want our baby to die of drowning in what's essentially a bucket?) and the issue of organic weaning (him: my sister didn't do organic and the kids are fine/me: fuck your sister, pesticides might cause cancer, why would you want your baby to die of cancer?).

None of them major, insurmountable things, really, and all easily solved if I could just find the right article on Guardian. com to convince Rich.

But I didn't think it would be a great idea to have one of these rows in front of Gill.

Rich was mute, wide-eyed and clearly concerned I'd try to get my vagina out to break the building tension.

'Do you want a cup of tea, Gill?'

It did get me thinking though: *what kind of mother am I now?* I had previously decided, of course, to just continue being the same woman I'd been when I got up the stick, and the baby would be an add-on to this – very Lean In. But I hadn't factored in how I might feel about this child and how that would affect every move I'd make from here on in. I just wanted to be a really, really good mum to this miraculous creature.

We discussed feeding – '100 per cent breast, on demand,' Gill said as she scribbled on the form, so at least we knew what we were doing – and my work plans 'SAHM.' I nodded, even though I had no idea that meant Stay At Home Mum and I didn't really know what I'd do yet. I told her I wasn't drinking coffee or alcohol, or even using mouthwash, but she didn't write that down. Cow. Then she asked about sleep – where did the baby sleep, what did we wrap her in, where was her room? This prompted a discussion and we decided from the smug seat of two relatively well-rested adults, sleep training wouldn't be for us – we'd let her feed on demand and remain a relaxed baby. She obviously loved her sleep and she was far less demanding than we expected a child to be. Gill seemed to approve.

We didn't want to make it difficult for ourselves when thus far it had been ridiculously easy. We decided we would be the kind of parents who wouldn't shout or inflict the cruelty of leaving her to cry. That sounded bloody awful, especially when I read that babies who were left to cry had rocketing cortisol levels – they were 'stressed' at three months. Sleep-trained babies would probably go on to shoplift, fudge their taxes and murder people. Newborns were used to the dark, wet space in your belly and so crying at night, when they weren't squished or comforted by the sound of your heartbeat, was a natural cry for help. Rich and I agreed we'd always be there to give that help, of COURSE we would! The cry could be fear, sadness, stress or discomfort, and we'd obviously do anything to quash those feelings in our innocent little tiny girl. Imagine!

Basically immune to the new mum stereotype

What was really blowing my mind was how strong I felt my body had become over the past few days. *I'm feeding my baby, I'm awake a lot overnight, and yet I feel good.* I hadn't cried about anything except the state of my vagina and I hadn't suffered the exhaustion I'd been warned to expect. I was just coasting along like we were on holiday, luxuriating in the languid hours of cradling my baby and having nothing else to do. Bona fide hippy mum, boobs out, cooing, tranquil. It felt so good feeling her tiny warmth in the crook of my arm or on my chest. She slept so much and we were under the ridiculous illusion that it was down to us, not simply that she was choosing to sleep and was comfy enough to do so. It still felt like our choice as to when we cradled her and when we put her down. When she was asleep more than she was awake it was a rare treat to get to be with her and see her looking at us, and we nearly fought over having her for those moments, jostling into her eyeline so she'd fix on one of us as her favourite.

'I do worry she might be narcoleptic though, Rich, do newborns get that?'

His answer was a resounding NO but he didn't even sound annoyed, because he too was under the spell. *Interesting, maybe we'll be happier than we ever were after all,* I thought.

I was nicer though, too. Even to my mum who broke the 'no visitors' rule nine times in the first three days. She'd popped by under the guise of delivering more nappies, gifts from her friends and more massive pants she thought I might need. But I was so serene; I actually enjoyed her clucking around, taking the baby and smelling her head with the same enthusiasm I suspect she once had for a nice fat line of Charlie. She was relieved that I wasn't as moody anymore.

The baby still hadn't cried either – not once! If she stirred, I'd feed her and she would fall asleep again. Obviously for a while I had to lick my finger and put it under her nose to feel for the cool puff of air that would confirm she was breathing, listening intently to her snuffling to check for signs of impending death. But we got into a good routine of a quick feed, then I'd gently lower her back into the Moses basket at my side, checking for the sound of choking on her own vomit, and eventually pass out myself. The muscles on my right side were getting quite ripped from the swivel-action of lowering the baby into her cot, combined with the upright posture for feeding. I'd got into a rhythm, it was all working.

'My dad – your granddad – he used to say I was making a rod for my own back, picking you up every time you so much as whimpered.' My mum was round again, cradling the baby in her lap as I watched, beatific smile plastered on my face.

'I don't think he was right, of course, but I did have to pat you on the back for an hour every night until you were about five just to get you to sleep.'

'I literally don't give a fuck, Mum. Isn't that great? I just do what I feel like doing, and I don't give a fuck what anyone else thinks!'

… Oh no, wait! No, I'm not immune, actually

I had a little cry bang on schedule on day four, and am surprised that the Rules of Postpartum Motherhood apply to me – I was not immune after all. But the cry coincided with a repeat of *X Factor* so it could have just been that. What I should have realised was that those tears were the drip-drip-drip you always hear before the ceiling comes crashing down and your whole house floods. And sure enough the peace was officially broken on day five, when my milk came in. I had assumed that since she was feeding contentedly my milk had already 'come in' (directly into her mouth, in fact), but another of the NCT Facts About Parenting was about to hit me right in the tits. Suddenly, the brief, painless feeds and the four-hour sleeps were over. I had turbo tits, firing out hot milk faster than anyone could handle and she wanted to suck up every drop.

'FUUUUUUUUCK, MY TIIIIIIIITS!' I'd shout out, as the burning 'let down' happened, when I'd have to bite down on a muslin cloth or scream into a pillow. Imagine a thousand needles boring into your nipples and then entire breast. My nipples bled as I shifted her from one to the other and back again for what felt like hours at a time. She began to projectile spew after every feed as I basically water-boarded her with my giant fist-tits.

And I couldn't find any answers to my questions – should I sterilise my nipples, for example? I mean, we knew by then we should sterilise bottles if we wanted to use one, but what about my human breasts, sitting in the same bra for two days in a row, dribbling then crusting over …? Should I be alternating? But then once she'd drained one boob, she'd only half drain the second before puking everywhere, so should I then start the next feed on that same boob, or swap? Or just kill myself now and save us all the bother?!

Rich started taking notes – '12.10am, Left Boob 10 minutes, 12.28am, Right Boob 7 minutes …' Quite the page-turner. He lasted 15 hours and gave up – it was hard to keep track, especially when I'd taken to tucking her in my top and feeding her when I was on the loo.

I expected that at least my boobs would get more breast-like as the milk flowed – I'd never grown past the 'perky' stage (i.e. tiny tits) and obviously longed for full, almost pendulous breasts I could swing around. The new ones though were like massive, hard boulders, higher than before and lumpy, like a condom filled with apple crumble and sand. The veins rose in vivid blue over each round mound and my nipples got bigger and darker. Rich looked kind of interested as I hauled one out of its saturated sling but gagged when he saw how bruised and chunky it looked.

I had imagined the milk would come out of the end of the nipple, and only when activated by all the sucking, but actually it sprayed out of several locations, shooting across the room if the baby didn't latch on quickly enough, or simply pulsing inside my bra and quickly soaking several layers of clothing and often our entire bed. I started stuffing four breast pads into my bras at night, but still they would absorb their fill within an hour and I'd be soaking wet again. And if I was feeding from the right, the left would shoot out milk at the same rate, so I had to tuck an entire swaddle blanket into my bra to soak up the flow.

I had to wipe my tits down after every feed, lobbing pad after pad from my bed into the bin, missing most of the time so that there were dark rings of milk on the carpet. When it was time to empty the bin, the pads had turned green and furry. I only had to hear a baby cry for the udders to start twitching and then burning and then spraying; if someone brushed past me or worse, hugged me, they could count on starting off the squirts again. She puked left, right and centre, shat more times than I thought possible and if I wasn't leaking, she was – up the back, down the front – wee, poo, sick, dribble.

I had zero control and didn't want to go far from either the sofa or bed for fear of the inevitable flood, whether that would be my tits, her puking or the deluge of shit and piss. Deciphering milk from sweat and baby sick and dribble was impossible. I was constantly moist. I was swimming in bodily fluids. For days it was just constant feeding, washing, feeding, dozing, feeding, manic note-taking to try and work out if there was a pattern to all this mayhem, and then some more feeding. Rich fed me and reminded me to pee, but otherwise I did nothing but try to direct the constant flow of milk into the kid without drowning her.

'What the actual fuck is going on?!' I would whine to Rich, who would just consult *Your Baby: Week By Week* and reassure me it was all normal.

'FUCKING NORMAL, IS IT?! WELL, THEN THAT'S GREAT, I'LL JUST ENJOY THIS FLOOD OF SICK AND SHIT

AND PISS AND MILK AND SWEAT, BECAUSE IT'S FUCKING NORMAL! It's like I have diarrhoea in my boobs.'

I think my hormones *might* have started to spike again, at this point. Who knows?

Luckily I did get to watch a lot of TV, though. And I liked that people brought me things while I sat there. Sometimes I knew she'd finished feeding but I wouldn't own up immediately, often not until I needed a wee. But none of it looked how I thought it would look, I didn't look how I'd expected. My belly was still numb, my tits were agony and even my arms and back ached with all the lifting and swivelling.

Since the way you look and feel is obviously key to feeling yourself, to your identity remaining intact, I could feel that familiar old disorientation creeping back in now. Clearly, pregnancy had stretched and swelled my body out of all recognition – the only bit of me that looked vaguely familiar was my fingers, and even they started to swell in the final week. But I had expected that as soon as I'd given birth I'd have my body back to myself. It would deflate like a balloon, gradually fitting into the shape it had been before all this began and I would feel more like my old self. The truth was I needed to get to know this new body with its extra paunch and its sorely missed labia. Not to mention the fact that my breasts had been repurposed AGAIN to keep the child alive as its sole source of sustenance. From fun bags to milk bags in a day.

It was like a fight between my brain and body.

Brain: WOOHOOO, YOU'RE A FREE AGENT AGAIN; YOU'RE A FUN AND FABULOUS AND QUITE SEXY FREE AGENT WITH AN EMPTY UTERUS! WE COULD DO ANYTHING, THE POSSIBILITIES ARE ENDLESS! WE

COULD RUN, WE COULD DRINK VODKA, WE COULD
SLEEP ON OUR BACK, WE COULD –

Body: Hold it, sister. You're a mum now, stop being so crazy.
The tits are going to fill with lumpy cottage cheese milk until
they are the size of boulders and they will hurt and squirt
whether you lie on your back OR side. And you just TRY lying
on your front, or running or drinking or shagging. TRY IT,
BITCH!!

It reminded me of those moments as a teenager when your
body surprises you with its overnight mutations – you know it's
just a natural rite of passage but it still shocks the hell out of you.
The hair, the swellings, bee-sting tits, the aches, the spots. It
messes with your brain – you start to compare yourself to other
people, the rate you change. And you discover how your body
will look after years of wondering what kind of shape you'll
evolve into. Disappointing for me as I was gunning for an hour-
glass and instead was straight up-and-down and completely
boobless. But you're all in it together, you and your friends.
When you have a baby you similarly sit wondering what your
new body will look like – for me, AGAIN, will I finally get tits?

But you kind of go at it alone. And you're not all in it together
because your partner isn't going through it; your mates are most
likely not going through it. Plus, your body has a major responsibility this time round – not just about keeping you alive and
luring in a kid that looks a bit like Leonardo DiCaprio in certain
lights. It's about keeping a whole other human being alive and
well-fed. Also, as a teenager you're moving on to a phase you've
been dying to enter for years; when you're a new mum it's more
like you're ageing, heading ever closer to being OLD and DEAD.
So I felt the changes more acutely than when I was a teenager

– I'd had more time to get used to the status quo concerning my body this time round, about 10 years actually. I quickly realised I would have to learn to dress differently, I'd have to use my arms and boobs differently, I'd even have to walk differently. If I thought pregnancy had done a number on my sense of self, it was nothing compared to the adjustments I'd have to make once I was officially a mum.

We decided to bathe with our baby; holding her in the water seemed like the most solid way to avoid drowning or slipping. One night it was Rich's turn and as he gazed lovingly into her eyes, she smiled slightly.

'Oh my God, she's smiling, she smiled at me!'

I was understandably jealous, until I saw a brownness creeping through the water behind her. A stream of shit was spreading stealthily through the bath. I screamed, Rich screamed and bathtime was over. The beautiful moment was shot to, well, shit, and I couldn't stop laughing.

The next night, Rich got his revenge. As I was cradling our beautiful daughter in my arms, I heard him whisper, 'YES! IT'S HAPPENING!' and that familiar cloud radiated from her bottom in a puff of poo.

Sleep deprivation is a motherfucker

Then suddenly, all at once the tiredness hit me like a baseball bat aimed at my brain. With every night feed the tiredness was made stronger and more devastating by whatever was flooding through me when the milk came down and I risked slipping into a coma as my head lolled. I had to shake it from side to side or march my feet on the spot in bed just to keep myself awake. In the day I couldn't speak, my mouth was so slow and floppy. At night, I'd sit bolt upright in the middle of the night or burrow under our duvet, throwing pillows and breast pads at Rich as I went. Evidently I was looking for the baby who had slipped down under the duvet in my mind. Sometimes she'd crawled there or walked out of the room and fallen down the stairs, others she'd managed to climb up onto the windowsill and was tapping on the glass with her tiny newborn fingers. (Pretty scary, actually. Mental note: don't watch *Chucky* ever again.) But of course she was always in her Moses basket alongside me, sleeping soundly. In my panic I sometimes nudged the white noise machine and startled her awake. Oh, the irony of this gadget actually *waking* her.

Now, before I had a baby, I would have said I could survive pretty well with no sleep. I would say I function despite having a lot of late nights. From a young age at school I'd happily stay up 'til 3am doing homework, and at university without parents to point out the time I'd be out most nights, occasionally watching the sunrise before bedtime, eating stale bread and drinking red Fanta while some boy snoozed in my single bed. I'd have a quick snooze during a lecture, and get going again that evening for round two, fuelled by apple-flavoured VKs. Other than a pretty severe flu virus every September as I got used to the routine again, and a few bouts of cystitis, I felt – and looked – great. It prepped me well for the cycle of fashion parties and late nights in the office when I started working in magazines. I could still do my job the next day, firing on all cylinders if I'd managed the right balance of coffee and peanut butter on toast to get me through to 5pm. Sleep was not integral to my being, it was just a societal norm I observed because I knew I'd get a runny nose after too many late nights on the trot.

But until you have it stripped from you and are tortured by its total absence from your life, you don't realise just how sleep shapes who you are. Or rather that without sleep, you are a totally different person. And a bit of a dick, actually. When you lose sleep, you lose so much more. There's the loss of perspective, sense of humour, cognition, the ability to speak coherently, the ability to focus, concentrate and to work. Your libido is affected, even your sense of taste. Not sleeping properly severs your ties with who you are and who you want to be. It skews your self-awareness. So, if you're keeping score, that's 1. Unrecognisable body, 2. Loss of work, friends and social life, 3. Strange brainwash effect of hormones and then, 4. Sleep deprivation to just really strip back all my key components.

The lack of sleep was a brutal attack on my senses, both a sharp battering and a dull throbbing inside my brain. And so the new me I had been so pleased to discover started to go bat-shit crazy REALLY fast.

I didn't know which day it was or which time of year, so from now on the order in this book might seem a bit hazy. You know what? It was, it is, I don't know WHAT is going on at this point. Our baby could have been newborn, she might have been four or five months old. It's all the same. But to give some sense of perspective: Rich was still on paternity leave so it had only been a week. Yep.

One night I screamed because a giant spider was hanging above Rich's head. He screamed too (he is really scared of spiders) and I promptly faceplanted the pillow again. No spider, my brain made it up. But I DID have to put some cardboard boxes on our windowsill because a bird kept flying into our room and scaring the baby. WAIT! NO! That didn't even happen! Did it? Nor did I have sex with my R.E. teacher from high school, but I became fairly convinced that I did and had to conceal the great shame from Rich and my baby, who would definitely be quite judgemental. *Did I have sex with him? It's possible. Or else that was a VERY vivid dream.*

'Rich, look, look, there are some little legs on the road! Over there, look!'

'What the hell are you talking about?'

'Can't you see those little legs in the road? They're like … maybe they're artificial limbs?'

'Do you mean those traffic cones?'

'Oh. Yes. Well, there *were* legs there, anyway. Maybe they've just … wandered off.'

I ached with tiredness, but would get wild bursts of energy, enough to ball the tiny socks she wore for maybe 10 seconds each day before they were kicked off into a corner. There were several pairs under our sofa – basically sleeping bags for dust bunnies – because neither of us could add picking up socks to the endless to-do list. The adrenalin was gone, the milk-sweats were draining me of any energy I had left and the baby bubble phase of paternity leave was about to end.

While Rich was making the most of all the time off – he was not pinned under a baby for the most part of the day, after all – I was becoming one with the sofa, its cushions permanently reshaped by my slumped body. Rich started working out in the afternoons with an *Insanity* DVD, jumping around and sweating profusely while I sat and watched with a bag of crisps.

I would stand in front of my wardrobe, slack of jaw and fanny, considering what one item of clothing would inflict the least amount of pain on my highly sensitive skin. I think this could be why fleece clothing does so well among parents. Because in every other respect it is a daft thing to wear when you have a kid – it exacerbates sweatiness, not to mention the fact snot and spit crusts up on that stuff like the top of a macaroni cheese. Stupid. But to be cocooned like that in something so soft you can barely feel it touching your skin, that's everything to a tired person. My eyes throbbed, my skin burned and my throat was constantly stuffed with lumps that threatened to ugly-cry me into a frenzy.

We didn't schedule feeding; I just did it on demand, because the health visitor had written it down already without trying to talk us out of it. And because you can't make any sensible or coherent decisions when you're THAT TIRED, we just carried on like that, thinking it was set in stone that we would parent in this vein forever.

'SHE SAID 100 PER CENT BREAST, IT'S 100 PER CENT BREAST!' I'd wail when Rich suggested we make use of the 16 baby bottles we had stashed in the kitchen.

'And we don't have a steriliser! What, do you want her to get fucking E. coli or … like, a dust disease?'

I did get a hand pump but after an hour of pumping I'd only managed a dribble, my hand was in a permanent claw and I was exhausted. It was so much easier to just sit there and let her do all the hard work. It was all too much for me to deal with when I didn't *need* to do it. I think formula is actually a marker for a capable and clever person who can add up and clean things properly.

We also bought a teddy with an in-built white noise machine, a glowing sheep, a new mattress, various sleep bags, swaddles and books – so many books – anything to try and fix this shit-storm.

I was in Japanese terms 'inemuri' – asleep while awake – according to *The Sleep Revolution* by Arianna Huffington, which confirmed that sleeplessness is linked to depression, anxiety, poor health, poor cognitive function. Guys, it could kill you! An Australian study which Huffington cites, proved that being awake for more than 19 hours at a time can cause a cognitive impairment equal to a blood alcohol level of 0.1, the point at which you're considered legally drunk. And there I was driving our child around, and without a left-side wing mirror, too. I was parenting while pissed up.

Much like a drunk person, I was very emotional, mainly over the probable demise of mankind. Whereas before I had my baby the selfish section of my brain was probably the biggest, now my empathy levels were rising scarily fast. Before the baby, if I didn't want to do something, I wouldn't do it. If it was an inconvenience to me, it probably wouldn't happen. But when my cervix effaced to allow my baby out of me, it let all the empathy creep inside me. I was not only subsumed with thoughts of my baby's wellbeing, but all babies and children. That's not my way of saying women who don't have kids haven't felt this way or that they are less empathetic, by the way, it's just that I personally wasn't *as* empathetic. I remember reading Charlie Brooker saying it was like a veil had been lifted when he'd had his baby, suddenly all the world's ills were visceral, and that's exactly what I've experienced as a mum.

I couldn't unsee or ignore other people's pain, I had to cry and fret and imagine it's my child in that position, that it's my pain and her pain. I refused to watch films about child abuse, cancer, dying parents or kids, missing kids, sad kids. I developed a severe Unicef habit, texting them every time I saw the posters, donating away the last of my paltry state maternity pay. I raged at the news, I'm saluting magpies to fend off this all-consuming sadness but to no avail, weirdly.

I was sad about the big things, falling like Alice in Wonderland down a rabbit-hole vortex of Facebook threads on childhood cancers, but also the fact that our daughter will probably not experience Saturday night on the sofa watching *Blind Date* with my dad, or the thrill of choosing a video from Blockbusters when she has tonsillitis.

I had never been more politically engaged, but I was also pissed up of course, so I was inarticulate and could only read the headlines and then I would lose my train of thought. I couldn't regurgitate the arguments that had won me over because I couldn't remember anything for longer than 30 seconds. I couldn't debate but I shouted CHILDCARE! HEALTHCARE! SOCIAL CARE! PUBLIC SERVICES! HELP!! like a militant goldfish.

I was also increasingly unreasonable – more correlations could be drawn with being hammered. I insisted on doing the night feeds alone (well, thanks to Rich's total lack of functioning mammary glands I couldn't very well have it any other way), but I didn't do it gracefully because I resented his deep sleep.

'THIS IS FUCKING OUTRAGEOUS!' I'd whisper-scream as I flounced out of bed to tend to our baby again, convinced it was somehow Rich's fault she was hungry/wet. It definitely couldn't be her fault – sinless little angel from the heavens – and it sure as fuck wasn't mine. The anger always abated as soon as I held her in my arms, but I'd return to bed seething, hopping mad. I looked and usually found a reason for her waking that could indeed be assigned to Rich, selfish Rich. If you're doing everything by the book and the kid *still* won't sleep, someone must be to blame. The main reason I found was when the door between the bottom of the stairs and our kitchen was left open when he came up to bed. I was convinced that the cold air from the kitchen would snake up the stairs, around the corner and across the hallway into our room, stirring her from her sleep. Either that or he hadn't put the nappy on properly. Or had distracted *me* from putting it on properly. Or he hadn't bought the next size up of nappies LIKE I'D SUGGESTED ONCE (though possibly just to myself). I was convinced he was lazy. And such a dick.

He was patient, though I did notice his teeth had begun to clench. *Maybe he's forgotten I gave birth out of my fanny and is starting to judge me by normal human standards*, I thought to myself. But still, he remained calm throughout my insane ramblings and teary shouting.

'It's really hard, Mum,' I tried my best not to cry as she held the baby in one arm and put the other around my shuddering shoulders, 'How did you cope?'

'I didn't, darling! It was fucking horrible! Your father was useless, despite having had six kids with his first wife, so we rowed all the time and I had nobody to turn to, and then he was either on tour or filming up north! My friends were all working, my mum was dead, and so I was all alone and miserable and hated life. It was BLOODY AWFUL!'

I had stopped crying. This comforted me in some way. It was just hard on everyone – deal with it.

Rich leaves us

OK, he goes back to work. He didn't have to change at all, really. Looking back, he agrees that having a baby had zero effect on his career.

Granted, by this point I disliked him intensely at night, but during the day he was the only thing holding it all together, making it possible for me to just feed and eat, feed and eat, on a continuous loop. He was endlessly patient with my mood swings, keeping his distance just when it counted most, and being so tender and gentle with my baby. *OUR* baby, sorry – I do that a lot. Not fair, is it? But I felt like I was doing the lion's share purely because of the feeding. And now, his part in this was over, and he was allowed to go back to real life, popping back into the brutal yet beautiful new bubble at home. Brutiful, if you will. That last Sunday was deliciously slow and cosy as the baby napped on us and we didn't get up from the sofa except to top up our cups and plates.

My first concern was, what would happen when I needed to pee? Would I wait until she was asleep then carry the Moses basket into the bathroom? It didn't seem very sanitary given the size of our bathroom meant she'd be very close to the loo wherever I put the basket. Would I be able to cradle her while I wee'd? Or worse? What's the point of sterilising everything in sight if actually you're then going to dangle her over a toilet filled with your own defecate?

A more pressing thought was what seemed like a daily visit

to the weighing-in clinic in town, where the health visitors could check she's growing properly and I'm not feeding her solids etc. These appointments loomed in my diary because while we were doing very well, thank you very much, we were mostly tucked away in our little house, winging it. When faced with professionals in the field of keeping babies alive, I worried I'd be told I was doing it all wrong. Or that the reason she was so peaceful and undemanding at the moment was because something was VERY WRONG. *What if I don't KNOW I've got Postnatal Depression? Maybe I'm manic? Fuck. And I don't have Rich to bounce off; it's just me, totally exposed. I think I might be found out as the clueless reprobate I truly am.*

I had lost confidence in everything except changing nappies and stuffing my nipples into things. *What if I'm no good at all this without him?* I wonder. *What if he's been keeping us both afloat in his usual understated way, and what if I crumble without him there to underpin me?* And suddenly, without a job to return to, maternity leave was stretching out ahead of me, a potentially lonely prospect. Work was EASY compared to this!

Day one was pretty nice though, actually. He looked nervous as he kissed us goodbye and hovered for a moment in the doorway, as if he'd forgotten something. I sent him lots of pictures of me lying in bed, wearing actual clothes, hair freshly washed, baby sleeping. Having panicked about the end of paternity leave, I learned there's something rather empowering about NOT sharing the experience. I had to just get on with it and not discussing every move before we made it was liberating. I also discovered the deliciousness of inaction. We'd been so intent on

Being Normal for the past two weeks we'd actually been really busy and I was so tired. As I secretly lay around watching TV and stroking our baby I realised this isn't so bad after all, letting motherhood just kind of wash over me and make me still. There were no witnesses, who might point out I'd become the listless lump I'd sworn I'd never become. Because even on my arse I was achieving great things – this baby was alive and occasionally smiling (admittedly, mainly after a fart). I was nailing a very important job here, and nobody else needed to know I was doing it in front of the *Mad Men* boxset. I always thought I'd struggle because before I'd always been working or tinkering around on Twitter or DIY manicures. I couldn't bear 'dead time'. And yet now it was the best thing ever. *OHMYGOD, why would ANYONE go back to work?!* I thought, eating a slab of pâté between two Hobnobs because I needed lots of fat and calories for all the feeding.

I went to all the various weighing sessions and nobody suggested I was doing a crap job. They were all happy I was breastfeeding and she was putting on weight in line with that daft graph that counts for nothing except whether you've managed to hold a naked newborn still enough on what looks like a kitchen scale before they shit all over it.

Once those appointments were over I'd have no idea what time it was, what day it was, and having counted down the days until I'd be a singular agent again, my baby and I were morphing back into one again. When left alone we were basically one thing and comfortably so. We were never apart and physically joined most of the time, thanks to the endless feeding. Looking back, once the shock had died down and I developed all the coping mechanisms for handling the turbo tits, it was the happiest I've ever been. It was blissful, being in a huddle with my baby, where I didn't have to consider much beyond the next nappy.

Of course soon the mess started to mount. I had things to do. All other mums would be cooking supper, cleaning the house, probably even dishing out BJs when the immaculately made bed was turned down. I had always insisted on sharing out the domestic duties in our previous life – I refused to make them my remit when we both worked and both had arms – but suddenly it felt like if I was going to stay home all day, I should be taking it all on. So tiredness not only robbed me of my get-up-and-go, it also took away my feminist stance on chores. I hadn't ever found any pleasure in keeping house and would absolutely shirk it all wherever possible. I had never ironed, I didn't polish things. Except my nails. The cleaning was squeezed into the hour before someone was due to arrive. I was used to never having my own time, and if there were enforced no-work moments, they usually contained alcohol or illness. What should I do? I was too tired to read – the words started jumping over one another and I re-read the same passage four or five times before nodding off. I couldn't exercise because I didn't want to. I was basically too knackered to do anything, but doing nothing felt so wrong. I should have slept, of course, but for some reason, that didn't sit well with me either. Given my time again, I'd lap it up, sleep for hours and hours; I wouldn't think twice. But I was reluctant and I *still* don't know why.

What did I do all day? I wondered when Rich asked. I couldn't remember. I started texting him in-depth lists of my achievements, and then I took to verbal vomiting all over him the minute he got home from work. Rich didn't always want to hear the minute-by-minute breakdown of our day, of course. But if I didn't tell him all the small things I'd done that day it was as if they never happened and I'd achieved nothing. So he disappeared to the loo for a good 20 minutes, and I would stand outside, shouting about the new combination of stain remover I'd tested out on the White Company babygro – you know, the one with the circus print, the little seals? – after the third up-the-back-shit-storm explosion of the day. Or was it the fourth …

The trouble was, there was no break in the mundane. We didn't socialise as much as we'd expected to because HELLO, WHERE ARE ALL OUR FRIENDS AT?! Plus, we were socially inept due to the sleep deprivation. Whereas I used to work from morning until evening, with an occasional lunch break in the middle, and then could unwind during the evening and sleep as I chose, now there was no break and no gap. No change from morning to noon to night. No timetable. There were fewer novel experiences once the feeding and nappy-changing was down pat, so the hours seemed to go so slowly. 'The hours are long but the years are short!' retorts an elderly aunt when I say it feels like it's been the longest month in the world.

I felt so boring and yet the words kept coming. I felt the domestic drudgery I was subsumed by was demeaning simply because of the way it'd been demeaned by the people around me. I mean, should a feminist take pleasure in successfully getting a shit stain out of the carpet, or managing to do a super-market shop and only forgetting seven items? On the one hand I struggled being the stay-at-home-mum because it was some-thing I'd railed against from an early age, and on the other I was loving parts of it because it was for this incredible child, it was for love. *Um, actually those kind of mundane things are THE ESSENTIAL UNDERPINNINGS OF LIFE,* I began to reason, but just as I thought it, I'd forgotten it again. I had applied the kind of standard I would never have applied to another mother (but isn't that always the way?) – if any of my friends had detailed this kind of day I would have been impressed. But I felt like my old self wouldn't have stood for this kind of shit. It felt like I'd gone from a pregnancy that was all about me – well, in my head anyway – to motherhood, which was all about someone else. It should have been called babyhood. And while I was loving it, I could definitely feel myself slipping away, the woman behind the baby.

I needed to go out. The first time, I couldn't put the buggy up once I'd got into town. Even when I'd mastered that in our living room though, I realised the equations that would produce an alfresco experience were mind-boggling. *First, I'll pack the nappy bag. OK, muslins, wipes, nappies – wait, has she had a shit yet? Is one due? Should we wait 'til she shits, possibly until tomorrow, or hope we can find a changing table somewhere? Where has a changing table in the loo? One where you're unlikely to catch herpes? And which outfit can be easily removed and reapplied? How many of those outfits will I need? What if she shits in the pram? Will I throw it out? Should I wrap her in towels, or hey, what about plastic? Cling film might keep the shit in? Oh look, she's shitting already. OK, I'll change her. Oh, and her entire outfit. OK, that's fine, that only took an hour. Now, should I feed her before we go? Where will I feed her once we're out? Hey, what if she needs a feed in the car, while I'm driving? Will I pull over?*

This took around three hours, and once I finally arrived in town I had no change for parking, so I drove home again.

Tits out

If I did make it out of the house, I was alone. And then she needed a feed. Now this was strange because I'd been brought up to NOT get my tits out in public. The first time it happened I was wearing a regular T-shirt and had to lift it up, despite the fact my entire jelly-belly was on show. This was more disturbing than the dripping nipple, to be honest. I grabbed a muslin and covered us both with it, so I was a mound under a sheet, jostling around as I tried to get the latch right. The next time I was properly dressed in something I could let down on just one boob, so all that was revealed was the nipple, and actually the baby did a pretty good job of concealing the whole thing with her mouth. *Great work, kid.* Mostly, people averted their eyes, or a kindly waitress would bring you water. Sometimes another mum would nod and smile, otherwise it was eyes down, get it done. It felt weird to feel the wind on my nipples, but it amazes me how quickly I got used to it. I'm also soon used to bending down to swab up puke from the floor, and perfected the art of looping a giant swaddle muslin through my bra strap so it acts like a little canopy, hiding your breast. I hear now it's not recommended – *by covering the breast, aren't you suggesting it needs to be covered, that the act of breastfeeding is not the beautiful, natural privilege it is?* No, dude, I'm just trying not to squirt your boyfriend in the face with my giant sprinkler nips and also, keep them warm.

Nobody ever criticised me, nobody seemed to care really. Slightly awkward when you see a male friend, interestingly, but even then – needs must. You just get on with it.

'They're not MY breasts anymore, so it's not embarrassing,' I explained to Rich one evening. 'Even the nipples are different now. It's like I've got comedy tits strapped on, and you can't be embarrassed about comedy tits.'

I'm not sure anyone understood this logic, but at least I was not housebound.

The only problem with this demand-feeding was that I couldn't go more than 10 feet from my baby. We were inextricably linked, I was her only source of sustenance for six months. I wouldn't get my body back then, after all. It would be a dairy farm system for nourishment, hydration and comfort.

Rich is a dick

I resented Rich slipping back into his old life so swiftly, making his way in the world outside, drinking coffee and talking to other people with such ease. Although of course I did not fully understand this at this stage – I was just aware he was REALLY pissing me off and made me want to say snide things to him. His body was the same, he looked the same, he wasn't leaking from what felt like every orifice. He was dealing pretty well with the sleep deprivation too – he fell asleep on the sofa a lot and there would be one day a week where he would be a bit short-tempered, but that was my only clue that he was a bit tired.

Simultaneously, I wanted to do everything for our kid because I was so in love, but I was tired and wanted him to do stuff, too. He couldn't feed her, granted. But he could change her, he could wind her, there was stuff he could do. 'SOFUCKINGDOITTHENASSHOLE,' I eventually yelled in response to his kind offer. However, this didn't make me nicer, as planned. Like everything I've experienced as a mother, the less you do, the less you want to do. I honestly believe if I'd been left alone to bring up my daughter I'd have continued to do it all without flinching or shirking. I'd have been broke, and found years later, talking nonsense to a picture of a racoon, but it was only when help and intervention were offered that I became reliant on it, interestingly. And after being so kind to each other in the daylight hours, we both hit our tiredness wall at night and began to value our own sleep more than the other's. So, I took to lying.

'It's your turn,' I would hiss, 'I've been up with her five times already.' Not true but it just came out of my mouth.

'Grace, you have not been up once yet. She's fine, just wait a minute …' he'd slur as he drifted back off to sleep.

'IF I WAIT A MINUTE SHE WILL BLOODY SCREAM THE HOUSE DOWN! YOU HAVE A WINDOW OF 20 SECONDS, THEN SHE'LL NEVER GO BACK TO SLEEP!'

'OK, OK, I'll get up, I'll just …'

'GET UP GET UP GET UP GET UP!'

'FINE!'

This happened pretty much every night, and every morning I'd pretend to sleep through her gurgling, fake a snore and a lip-twitch so he'd get up. Even though he had to be at work in another hour. But if he even coughed …

'I'VE BEEN UP ALL NIGHT, DICKHEAD! YOU HAVE BEEN ASLEEP THE WHOLE ENTIRE TIME!'

I don't think I actively loved him anymore. Or at least, not consistently. All the things I'd fallen in love with – the slow, measured voice, acerbic humour, his endless patience – were now insurmountable flaws that made him a terrible parent. And the worst thing was he was actually being a brilliant parent, which only served to make me feel more insecure and crap as a mum.

One night very nearly lead to divorce proceedings, for him on the grounds of irreconcilable differences, and for me on the grounds THAT HE WAS AN IDIOT.

I'd taken the baby into her nursery across the hallway to change her nappy, our second default position to get her back to sleep when feeding didn't work. I had just one eye open, thinking it would be easier to get back to sleep if I didn't fully come to. I had unpopped her onesie, removed her nappy and was just lifting her legs by the tiny ankles to slip a fresh nappy under her bottom when, 'PPPPPPRRRFFFFFFFFFFFT!' She shot a stream of liquid poo up in a perfect arc, which splattered all down me. It was like the machine guns that shoot out cream in *Bugsy Malone*. I was covered from head to waist, and as I paused to consider what to do, I felt it drip off my chin onto my nightie. Another fart sounded and I ducked; she hit the wall behind me with a Jackson Pollock-style splatter of digested breast milk.

'RICH! RICH! RICH!' I bellowed as I lowered her legs, not knowing what to do first – clean her, clean me, clean the room …

I called out at least another 10 times before he stumbled out of our room, his eyes still shut, mumbling about already getting up twice before.

'SHE HAS SHAT … EVERYWHERE!' I screamed at him, doubly irritated at his slowness.

'NO, SHE HASN'T, SHE HAS NOT,' was his reply. 'I can't see any shit, she has not shat.'

'OPEN YOUR FUCKING EYES, MORON,' I bellowed again, realising he was still asleep.

He was adamant I was making it up, and so eventually I sent him back to bed, taking on my other exhaustion-related alter ego, the martyr. *I'll just do it my bloody self then, shall I?* I seethed through gritted teeth, as I pulled the throw off the armchair and placed it and then the baby on the floor. I used a whole packet of baby wipes to clean the wall, the floor, myself, the baby and cursing myself for insisting on the water-only Wet Wipes that contained zero cleaning agents and so were useless on a shit-covered wall and carpet. I took all my wet clothes off and stood shivering in my pants as I quickly cleaned the one dribble of poo off my daughter's leg, dressed her and placed her in her cot for a minute, while I gathered the throw, my clothes and her clothes into a bin bag and used the poxy water wipes to clean myself. I could have showered of course, once she was safely in her cot, but I was not thinking straight at all at that time, and faced with an actual shit storm you compromise on your hygiene laws. Eventually I returned to bed and returned the baby to her Moses basket, huffing and muttering as I did so to no effect since Rich was already deep into an REM cycle and dribbling onto his pillow.

In the morning he denied all knowledge.

'Look, you're lying a lot at the moment, aren't you? In your sleep? We all get a kick out of it, it's pretty funny, but you can't be mad at me because of a made-up poonami.'

'I'm not fucking lying! OK, I may have lied in the past – whatever – but this time it's honestly true!'

I had done such a good clean-up job, there was little evidence, but I pulled the nightie I'd been wearing out of the bin bag and thrust it in his face.

'HA! See?! Shit.'

He dry-heaved and asked me not to do that again.

All I wanted was for him to tell me I was doing a good job, even when I was acting like a psychopath.

I argue now that I had a smaller amount of kindness in my being and it all went on my kid. I misdirected a lot of rage at Rich, but also at my mum and anyone who attempted to give me advice, like, 'Have you tried a bedtime routine?' or, 'Try reading a book at bedtime, it works for us every time.' To be fair, those are pretty stupid things to say to someone who has clearly tried everything. *Oh no, we just fling her on the floor most nights with a KFC Zinger Tower to calm her down.* But also now I've had a bit of sleep (a *Bit*), I know I was unduly mean, hissing and spitting at everyone any time I felt maligned or patronised. I was wracked with self-doubt and the conviction that it was my fault she wouldn't sleep.

I am a dick

So 12 weeks in, I'd lost it. I was used to being brain-dead most of the time, used to feeling foggy and sore all the time. *This is just how it is,* I thought, unsure as to when babies started sleeping and too tired to find out. The acceptance of our lot was sugar-coated by the beaming baby who – when awake – just dolled out loving smiles at all hours. I was so happy. And every evening I was hopeful that a change was coming. I was fine so long as nobody questioned me. Great time to visit the in-laws for a long weekend, I'm sure you'll agree. In-laws, unless you're the exception to the rule, will always be on hand to support your self-doubt and of course, back your husband's every move.

We took her up north to meet everyone in the depths of a dark and cold winter and the sleep deprivation was just starting to throb between my eyes. I called my mother-in-law the week before to ask please could we just stay at home while we were with them and could we keep it quite low key because we were all knackered. She agreed, although of course the nephew and niece would be popping in, and the aunties and uncles were coming up from the surrounding towns. And Liz from next door was stopping in for tea.

After five hours of crawling along motorways and stopping to stretch and feed (I was very conscious a newborn shouldn't be in a car seat for longer than 1.5 hours at a time and inwardly felt this whole episode was basically child abuse, so I was already in a really good mood before we'd set foot in their house), we made it, and were ushered into a house full of people.

The baby was taken off me as soon as we stepped out of the car and I felt my stomach lurch as she was passed around and around, Liz-next-door stumbling in at some point in her dressing gown to get a look. I sat in the dining room, quietly lactating into my bra. And that feeling I should have had watching our family coo over our awesome kid never came – I just felt anxious. What if she didn't like it? It all smelt different, there were so many strangers. Shouldn't I be feeding? Everything felt brighter and sharper, my eyes stung. Rich eventually swooped in and took the baby and me upstairs to feed – something I was usually happy doing in front of anyone – but I needed to be out of the spotlight, away from the comments on how I was doing it. I held her close and let her feed until she slept, then just sat there, staring at her, stroking her little hand. I know it was self-ish – this was her family and they didn't get to see her often. I knew how precious and brief this time was and how they deserved to soak up every second with her, but I couldn't move. It felt like putting her out in the circus to be watched and poked and prodded. I was so angry, even in the midst of these people who wanted nothing more than to love and enjoy our baby. My mother-in-law shouted up the stairs, 'Are you nearly done? Mandy's here with the kids.' I snapped, and bellowed down, 'I'LL COME DOWN WHEN SHE'S FINISHED!' and then cried for half an hour.

I used these feeds to escape and be quiet and alone for a minute – alone with the baby. So I fed her A LOT.

'But you just fed her!'

'Well, she needs a sleep now otherwise she'll be wired by bedtime.'

'You're not tired, are you, sweetheart? You don't want to nap, do you? You want to stay up with me and play!'

Rich and his family are very much from the 'well, it never did me any harm' camp, whereas my family are the founding fathers of the 'shit, we're all going to get cancer and die!' school of thought. So I think for the most part they think I'm stark raving mad.

The thing is, our families both just wanted us to be happy and relaxed, and from the outside could see all the things we were doing to make life hard for ourselves. I should have said, 'Thanks for the advice, we're just going to try it our way for now.' Instead I said things like, 'FUCKING HELL, RICH, YOUR FAMILY THINKS I'M SHIT AT THIS!'

I was grumpy and resentful all weekend, driven to distraction by the clearing of pots and pans at 7am when we'd finally got to sleep, and the sound of the breakfast news at 9am, followed by late-night card games and whoops of delight from the other grandkids. Because, you know: happy people are the worst, aren't they?

'The routine, Rich, the routeeeeeeeeeen!' I'd cry hysterically, swaying regardless of whether or not I was actually holding a baby. Because the routine is all I had! It was how I knew what I should be doing at any one time, and when the next respite was due. Without it, everything was chaotic and scary. He kept telling me to relax, I kept wanting to cry.

We went into town to seek out strong coffee and a fight over who got to push the pram ensued amongst the cousins, until I marched up and took the handle from the lot of them, not content to see my baby bowling towards cars, pushed by a seven-year-old who couldn't yet see above the pram's hood. My mother-in-law was itching to push it too, but I could feel it and obstinately held on until my knuckles went white. Why was I such a bitch? It was half primal instinct, half a knackered, entitled thing, I think. I didn't even care about pushing the pram, usually! I was just a bitch, plain and simple.

The day we were going home I was brittle. I'd been awake most of the night, and between the 3am and 5am feeds I just lay there, looking up at the ceiling, cursing Rich's soft breathing and the slither of light coming in from above the curtain rail. The clock flickered to 5.09 and the baby slept on. *Oh, NOW you sleep in,* I thought. I was desperate to get up and go. As soon as she'd burped and puked all over the duvet, I leapt out of the bed and got our stuff together, told Rich it was time to go and crept downstairs to where my mother-in-law was already sitting in her dressing gown as the grandkids slept on the sofas.

'You're leaving already?' she asked, crestfallen, but I think caught my thunderous face and changed tact, 'OK, well, must just get a picture of all the grandkids together then.'

'Really got to get going before the traffic starts –' I started, but she took the baby and placed her in their laps while they rubbed their eyes in confusion.

'Do you think she'll wake up soon? It's just nicer for the picture if she's awake, isn't it?'

I picked up the baby and flounced out of the house. I sat in the back of the car with her, every so often taking off my belt to stretch across and stick my boob in her mouth while we drove, delirious, angry and illegal. WHY was I being so awful?!

CHAPTER SIX

3–6 MONTHS

Wow, I look weird. And my fanny is really weird. Actually, I feel weird too, in my brain. I am so tired, my tired is tired. Hmm. I do NOT know what I am doing. What am I doing?! Wait, where was I?

NOT losing weight

Once breastfeeding was assimilated into Things I Do Now – I'd done it in public, standing up and even on a packed bus – and it was no longer a blood-bath/novelty, I grew less aware of my tits and started to consider the rest of my body. Along with the rest of the world, apparently. Because what struck me was how much everyone talked about when I would lose the baby weight. Friends and family would routinely reference it in the same breath as 'how's she sleeping?' and 'how are you feeling?' 'Are you back in your jeans yet? Wow, you've dropped a bit since we last saw you? Hey, Spanx are great though, eh?'

The midwife, as she stepped over my blood pooling on the floor of the delivery room, told me breastfeeding would help (I hadn't asked), the health visitor cautioned me not to live off cake (I hadn't asked) and then the NCT girls started booking in group workouts and discussing jogger prams while I liked the sound of a stroller infinitely more. Strolling sounded mega. I hadn't asked ANY OF THEM for advice, but it was just accepted that it was something we'd all want to know about.

'Losing the baby weight' gets way too much airtime, so I'd sooner not address it, or just flood the pages with all the kind of stridently positive thoughts about how fabulous I felt and how empowered I was by the whole process of pregnancy and birth. *I love me as I am*! I crow, *I won't change for anybody*! Well yes, and no. Full disclosure: I felt a bit lost in this body. How I looked contributed to how different I felt now I was a mum. How MUM I felt. There were so many bits of me that were unrecognisable. So I chose to ignore it. Plus it didn't bother me that much because I felt like everything was still in a state of flux – who knew what I would end up with? I knew my belly wouldn't just suck itself back in like a whoopee cushion the minute my baby vacated the womb, but losing weight sounded a bit … premature. And I was too consumed with other things to make room for this concern at first.

As time went on, I was simultaneously being encouraged to fatten my baby up as quickly as possible and drop the odd pound that was keeping my midriff warm every time I had to lift up my top to feed. It's like a transaction must take place – baby put on weight, mum lose weight – and all at the same rate. Look, I like clothes that fit and being able to run for the bus without my thighs chafing as much as the next person, but lose weight?! I was just trying not to lose my mind.

Sorry, did I not just drop 7lb 9oz of baby weight out of my vagina? You also want me to make my arse … what, higher? Smaller?!

Maybe I should have been scoffing kale and cakes made from sweet potato (not a cake – that's a savoury scone at best, but basically, a pie)?! I don't think so! I wore leggings and a shirt or a massive jumper EVERY SINGLE DAY, so I wasn't worrying about what to wear. For the first time in my life, what I wore didn't matter to me, as long as my undercarriage was warm and I could get my tits out on demand. I was layering up, cloaked in coats and scarves. I was sitting down a lot. I honestly didn't really know what it all looked like underneath.

But when I did look down at my belly, now a soft, wrinkled paunch that literally hung between my hipbones, I struggled. Of course I didn't like it! It was like somebody else's body had eaten mine. In the bath, my breasts spread apart to nudge my arms and this belly wobbled in between. The stretch marks were like wrinkles rather than scars, so that below the smooth ridge of what were once upper abs, there was this old-lady-jowl flopping about in the water. My belly button was a huge hole in a ring of flesh – like a wet donut.

What I had to get to grips with was that the new belly wasn't 'mumsy' because there is no such thing as a motherly stereotype – we all have different bodies and to continually bastardise this word is to do all mums a disservice.

Originally, I'd grown this softly curved belly during the 90s, arguably the most unforgiving decade for the midriff. Crop tops, the knotted shirt, jeans slung so low you had to shave your entire bush off lest it peek over the top. Combat trousers that squeezed your love handles up and out like a sausage from its skin. And satin – satin going-out tops, dresses, all bodycon and skimming and squeezing. Belly buttons never look right under satin – innies look cavernous and outies look like hernias. I refused to be satin's bitch.

So at 16 I consciously honed my stomach by eating just Melba toast during the day and quite often burying my supper in the garden, come evening. I fainted a lot, I did 100 crunches a night. I smoked a bit to stave off the desire for a cheese sandwich, and I accidentally overdosed on probiotics until I shat through the eye of a needle. But no matter what, I still had a little curve under my belly button. It was punishing – flattening it, squeezing into knock-off Spanx from the market that left livid red marks across my hips. I spent hours putting on tops and taking them off again, scrutinising the way they sat over my belly, pinching and smacking the flesh. I WANT TO LOOK LIKE BRITNEY IN THE 'SLAVE4U' VIDEO, DO YOU NOT UNDERSTAND, YOU USELESS BIT OF SKIN? But ultimately I only ever showed off the burgeoning abs at the weekend since I was still in school uniform the rest of the time, and eventually gave it all up, taking instead to self-consciously placing a hand over my lower belly and wearing empire lines.

Just as my mum had warned me back then, I now look back on those days with a loving nostalgia for how smooth it was. Yes, it was curved more often than not, but it was so smooth. I should have shown it off *more* if anything.

So no, I didn't like this new wobbly belly or the stretch marks, which looked like I'd been savaged by Winnie The Pooh on crack, but I was more forgiving. Thanks to being knackered and the fact that this time my body had served a purpose. I started to think, *Yes, it's changed, but this is a grown-up softness, it has housed this most brilliant of kids. It has stretched and is probably unable to snap back now.* I was fairly sure that if the skin was permanently torn, the muscles were most likely shot to shit, too. I did want to feel less heavy (I don't mean when I jump on the scales – which I never have, never will – but when I lugged myself and my kid around, I wanted to feel strong and lithe and quick … Thinking about it, I could have just put the changing bag and the buggy down, couldn't I?). But, did anyone actually CARE what I looked like at this point?

I was lucky too that the kind of adulthood I felt like I'd been thrust into wasn't built in the image of supermodels, who for me are always frozen around age 21. In my head a beautiful adult woman was Kirstie Alley, Daryl Hannah, my high-school art teacher Miss Codd and my mum. All quite busty girls with solid thighs and arms who could swing at anyone who suggested they 'lose the baby weight'. I felt I had a good distance from the misogynistic nonsense of post-baby diets and the airbrushed models who lost 'the baby bulge' after two weeks of breastfeeding, probably because I've worked for magazines – I know it's all jiggery pokery behind the scenes, and not much of it is true enough to trust just with the naked eye.

The only thing that threatened to undo all this burgeoning body positivity was when I said to a friend's husband as said friend stood grinning at their baby something along the lines of, 'Doesn't she look great?!' And he replied:

'Yeh, but she's worked hard at it. You'll get there.'

Well, fuck me, I thought. *I don't want to work, I'm on bloody maternity leave. That's the whole point!* It hurt, because for the first time my own idea of how I looked – basically, fine – was called into question. I was aware that a lot of mums saw yoga and Pilates as much-deserved 'me time', but I did not. Ultimately, my body – like every other woman's – was still up for consumption and debate, but luckily I wasn't privy to it. From 'How you've grown!' as a kid to 'Is she sexy or not?' as a teenager, I was now entering the bit that comes just before 'Isn't she ageing well?', the bit where other people consider whether you're staying on top of things. But amazingly, after that initial sting I realised for the first time in my life, I didn't care. I thought, his opinion of how I look just doesn't matter. Imagine the worst – he's sat at home thinking I'm fat and lazy. Do I care? Does that really bother me? Will I mount a treadmill because he may or may not be thinking that? No. It just made me more determined that by the time my daughter had grown (or not grown) breasts, she wouldn't hear a single comment along the same lines, ever. I felt quite smug about this personal development, actually. I was a better person for this sense of perspective. I would still go wild when I couldn't snaffle up my belly into a pair of leather trousers, of course, but I didn't fear or dress up for other people's gaze, or long for their approval in the same way. GROWTH!

I didn't *just* care about how this issue affected me anymore, but ALL PEOPLE. I made a point of telling other mums how wonderful they looked, pointing out sparkling eyes, warm cheeks, a colourful scarf, ANYTHING, because I knew they too were often hearing, 'You look knackered!' and 'Oops, no longer eating for two though, are we?' Fuck that.

Obviously I put a picture of my jelly belly with all its stretch marks up on Instagram, because #millennial, but also in a narcissistic attempt to prove to myself that I didn't care anymore. I was in *control* of the consumption of my body. Of course the feedback was warm – they didn't want me to feel insecure, they wanted me to celebrate my body so they could celebrate theirs. It's like the snaggle tooth that jumped out of line as soon as my retainer came off, and the birthmark on my nose I've had since birth. It's there, why try to hide it?

The erupting mammary shelf

That said, I did do one exercise class, but just because I was peer-pressured into it. I was aware I'd declined one too many NCT meet-ups, so when one of them booked us all into a post-natal workout class, how could I possibly duck out? THAT'S when they'd finally all start partnering off into holiday-buddies and I'd be out on my arse, booking a one-berth caravan to share with the in-laws in Wales. I worked out that if I wore two pre-baby vests and two T-shirts over that I didn't wobble as much – I mean, I could barely fucking move, let alone wobble. We lined our babies up in their car seats and obeyed the trainer's orders, starting with a gentle jog up and down the room. *Totally got this,* I thought, *I think my tits might start bleeding soon but I feel quite strong.* As I ran back and forth I could feel the changes more keenly, as the boulder-boobs walloped around. My legs though, they were burning through, I felt strong and powerful. Until the third lap, by then I was dying. I managed to find a way out of the next class – 'I'm not bloody coming, it was awful!' – and I went back to sauntering my way through life.

Another group activity later forced me to confront my new body again. Three months in, the baby's swimming lessons started. Cue *JAWS* theme tune, because it had the potential to be horrific. And although I had misgivings about stripping down to the bare minimum in front of a room full of strangers (weird at the best of times), I couldn't let a potential body image crisis get in the way of her becoming a water baby, as planned.

Picking a swimsuit was a bit of an ordeal. To begin with, I thought I'd wear my pregnancy tankini but it was stretched out of recognition, like a metaphor for my body really – loose, flapping and a bit grey. But I used to work at *Vogue*, so you know – I know about shopping for clothes, right? I had some good underwear from M&S, so I went back and bought a black swimsuit with 'tummy control'. Controlling my tummy seemed like a good idea – the alternative presumably being it flopping free of its own accord.

But actually tummy control simply forced half my stomach skyward to join my tits, creating the impression of a mammary shelf beneath my chin. *OK, well, I'll be underwater*, I reasoned, *this is fine. And all the mums will be at the same stage having babies of the same age, so we're all in it together. Sisterhood, yeh!*

Except that it was all dads. Six dads and me. And my erupting mammary shelf.

Picture the scene – three months after giving birth, you're squeezing and folding your flesh into a swimsuit, sidling up to a swimming pool surrounded by strangers, with no hands to steady yourself, as you bravely hold your baby aloft, surreptitiously shielding that errant tit that just won't stay inside your suit. You wade in to what is essentially a warm soup of breast-milk and baby piss, and since swim-nappies are basically shit-tea-bags, potentially a fair amount of defecate on the side. As the dads studiously lifted their tiny babies in and out of the water in time with 'Old Macdonald Had a Farm', I just floated through a cloud of my own lactate, trying not to pee as the warm water dragged my bladder down to my knees. *I definitely think I'm going to prolapse something*, I thought, as the wading became more effortful and my insides took longer to bounce back up with the rest of me.

The real problem was getting dressed afterwards. They kept the changing rooms hot, so as soon as the pool water started to evaporate off you, you were cloaked in sweat. You try getting too-tight jeans up over your knees when you've got a sweat on, and a slippery, wet baby squeezed under your arm. The logistics alone blew my mind. It was when another mum was trying to wrestle my cheap, sticky nursing bra down past my shoulders and the changing room door swung open to reveal me and all my bits to the poolside spectators that Rich took over the swimming lessons ...

But I managed – the self-conscious and yet ridiculously beautiful 17-year-old me would have sooner DIED than been subjected to this kind of exposure. Even the 28-year-old me wouldn't have relished it. I didn't wear tight tops because I was convinced they didn't suit me, for God's sake. So I must have been growing up. Or you know, just too tired to care.

Ode to my broken vagina

There was one body part that wasn't so easy to ignore, though. My vagina was forever changed. And unlike a midriff, which is really only necessary for crop-top wearing, I NEEDED MY VAGINA TO DO STUFF! My six-week check-up (which I finally got round to attending at the eight-week mark) suggested my vagina might be ... neater than before. The nurse was keen to give me a smear test since I'm on the official watchlist for suspect cells and haven't had one for over a year, but she was unable to get even the smallest speculum in.

'I mean, this speculum was minuscule, and you have such a massive penis,' I tell Rich, stroking his ego so I won't have to stroke anything else. Four months into motherhood and I still had a pinprick sized opening down there. One morning, it all got a bit too much and I spilled my guts to Lou. We were in one of those bleak coffee shops in the middle of a shopping centre. Pre baby, these were my idea of hell, but now it shone out of the alienating maze of shops like a beacon of seats and lukewarm drinks.

Between us, Lou and I had about two thirds of one normal vagina left, thanks to the butchery of our respective labours. Having finally sat down, winched my kid into position under the now permanent fixture of the oversize muslin across my body, and settled all my belongings within reach, despite not being able to move inside my massive puffa coat, I realised my fanny was in a twist. Not a proverbial twist, it had folded and one bit had got stuck under the other like when you try to close an envelope without licking the sides. It really hurt. I shifted about, as well as anyone can shift with a four-month-old baby attached via a small yet increasingly long nipple. I was sweating and aching. I'd had enough.

'UGH, FORFUCKSSAKE! Mate, my fanny's all bloody twisted. GOD, IT HURTS!'

It's always a gamble, talking fannies with a new-ish friend, but she moved in closer,

'Yep, me too. Actually …' both of us squeezed our babies to our chests as we jiggled towards one another, 'I'm going to have a fanny op.'

'WHAT?! Like a designer vagina?'

'No, a NORMAL vagina. I've been emailing a friend who's a gynaecologist in London and she says they've made a right mess of my fanny. I'm going to have it all sorted out under general.'

'And how does she know it's a mess for sure?'

'I emailed her pictures.'

'YOU EMAILED HER PICTURES OF YOUR FANNY?!'

'Yeh – dead easy. Just used the iPad with the camera bit facing me. I felt like some sort of vlogger.'

'What email address did you use?'

'Just my work one.'

'You used your work email address to email someone photos of your vagina? I don't think you should do that, Lou.'

'I hear what you're saying. But at least my fanny is going to be properly nice after this. I'll be able to sit on Formica work-tops without screaming.'

When I pictured an episiotomy, I figured there was a tiny slice in the inner bit of your vagina that made the exit a bit wider. A cut made with a scalpel. Like, if your knicker elastic is a bit tight and you give it a little snip so you can breathe. So once the head was out, you'd be able to just stitch that little line up again – a scar UP INSIDE YOU which nobody would ever notice and you're back to being fanny-fabulous. NOT SO. When you're at full stretch and the kid's head is crowning, it's actually all the *outer* stuff that's acting as a crown (the clue is in the name), and so when a registrar approached my fiery loins with a pair of scissors, she meant to chop my labia. Rich saw her, he said it was as if she was cutting a really tough bit of meat because of the effort she had to put in. Great.

At first, the whole thing was just so swollen and bruised (I'm told – I didn't have a look myself because I thought it might hurt more if I knew how beaten-up it looked) it was hard to tell what I had left down there. I sensed a chunky bit to one side, which was thick with stitches and scar tissue. A while later it became clear something was missing. On one side my labia was the same as ever, a young person's labia, I thought. On the other side, it stopped abruptly halfway down. WHERE DID IT GO? I feel sad thinking about it sitting in some kind of vat of human waste in the hospital, alongside dirty appendix and maybe a foreskin or two. Do you think it was incinerated? That makes me so sad.

Lou did get hers re-stitched but there was no such makeover for my besmirched fanny. It's been forever altered but now it's not actually painful (bar the odd bout of phantom flap pain I get in mourning of the bit they chopped off). I feel like it's just entered another bit of its life cycle, where it's not as … pretty. Wait, was it ever pretty, though? It's been through so many little milestones, I've tried to consider this latest butchery as just another stitch in the rich tapestry of a vagina's life. Although don't mention stitches around it because it'll fold up on itself again like a hedgehog.

When I was a tiny girl, I paid very little attention to my vagina. I didn't experience my first frisson of pleasure until I was about 10 and I accidentally sat on a Barbie, and even then I didn't think to explore that further. When swimming with my school friends, we sometimes used to queue up at the water filter and let it blast against our nether regions, quite unaware we were ostensibly getting off in front of the whole leisure centre. But otherwise – not interested.

I suppose the fact that I couldn't really see it in great detail facilitated the near total lack of acknowledgement I gave my vagina, the thing I assumed was only useful for urinating. I didn't scrutinise it like the rest of my body, and when the time came to consider letting boys see it, I assumed it was just your run-of-the-mill, bog-standard vagina. It worked well enough, I guess. I did go through a phase experimenting with pubic topiary after a boyfriend suggested I might have a trim, but the lightening strike I tried to create using a stencil cut out of a Shreddies box was crap, and I decided to stick to a short back and sides. A nod to my womanhood with a smooth (if not slightly itchy) surround, not unlike a marble fireplace.

Years later, I'd have one abnormal smear after another and suddenly that whole area – or the cervix anyway – was a hotbed for potential cancer. I was just a bit scared of it. I'd had a whole chunk of innards removed with an electrically-charged wire (like a super-specific fetish, right there) – AKA a LLETZ procedure to remove suspect cells and to prevent cervical cancer developing – and it had been OK ever since. Though it wasn't entirely pleasant, I couldn't see a single hint of this inner trauma on the outside. Nothing about the way it looked or felt had changed through any of these duff experiences.

Then it had to suffer a stretch of over 10cm, a head and then a body using it as a thoroughfare, and a pair of scissors lobbing bits of it off onto the floor. It was such a bloody battle, my vagina was officially war-torn. And unlike the previous occasions it had suffered an injury, this time it was very important to me. It was this thing I needed for sex, a key part of my connection with my husband. With all the changes we'd been through as a couple, the vagina was the familiar constant which harked back to our youth in many ways, the heady days before we had jobs or mortgages or anything really. It was the bit of me that was always young and about pleasure, while the rest of me had to mature and handle responsibility. Plus, I'd had it for ages and I knew where I was with this vagina.

Now it was changed and repurposed. Extraneous bits (which, by the way, were not extraneous but full of nerve endings) had been removed, and anytime anyone looked at it they'd know something had occurred, if not specifically that a baby had been born out of it. I recently heard psychotherapist, Philippa Perry, say on Radio 4 that our genitals, our sex, are 'the very core of our selves'. If that's the case, bloody hell, it might explain some of the annihilation my self went through.

Sex is OUT of the question

Might be nice though, I imagined Philippa saying, *a nice little bit of sex is just what the doctor ordered! A sweaty orgasm, that'll make you feel like your old self.* Firstly, with all due respect (LOVING your work), are you FUCKING MAD, Philippa?! And secondly, did you not hear the bit about my broken fanny? My sexuality was up in there, in that mutilated vagina. Also, my sexuality being another facet of my identity that I associate with being young, I suddenly felt old. 'Past it' had never seemed so apt – that boat has sailed, the boat where I experiment and flaunt myself and fully utilise the power of sex. And have a pretty vagina. My sense of humour, my dress sense even … I knew my sexuality played a huge part in all that I was. But I felt asexual more than anything else, like my sexual desire had fallen out of me along with the placenta. I was spending 24 hours a day being a mum and I couldn't see where sex would fit into this new identity. Well, it absolutely didn't fit actually, because I'd been stitched up too neatly.

At that time, I had very little personal space. I was feeding on demand and since we didn't have room for a baby bouncer, she was always around or on me. In fact I've never really gone back up to full capacity – nowadays I'm climbed on, puked on, followed constantly and occasionally slept on. But back then when she was a tiny baby I encouraged her to attach to me like a limpet. It meant feeding her was a doddle, it made me feel good and it didn't give her a single opportunity to cry or grizzle. I sweated, I ached, I bruised, I itched.

If you've been holding your baby for 10 of the past 12 hours, the gentlest of shoulder squeezes can send you into a snarling rage.

'Don't touch me!' I'd yell, even if Rich hadn't yet tried to. It was as if all my physical energy was tied up in my child and so I had nothing left to give.

I fully appreciated during more lucid hours that this was tough on Rich. I was a different person all over again, obsessed with my baby and with room for nothing else. I offered him zero physical affection and had no time to listen to him. He came home from a day of dealing with people in pain and suffering, had a five-minute car drive to unwind, and then was faced with a slightly rancid-smelling woman and her boring stories. But I couldn't put another person's needs before my own, having spent all day denying every natural instinct for self care to keep our daughter alive. As for sex? I was not to be touched unless it was by a healthcare visitor or to be milked in between feeds. So that's how it went for a while. He was kind and unerringly patient, but ultimately spent longer and longer in the loo doing *Extreme Sudoku.*

Four weeks into parenthood I gave him a cheeky blowjob because I felt so bad about the lack of intimacy and this new half-life he was being forced to live, and it seemed like the only anatomically viable way to reinstate the relationship we'd enjoyed for the past eight years. I want to say I did it for me too, and I did like remembering that side of my psyche, but ultimately there wasn't much in it for me. I knew I was simply adding it to the list of things I had to do that day to keep all my humans happy. THAT IS SO DARK AND AT ODDS WITH MY SEXUAL ETHOS, GUYS.

On the upside, I had a story. After weeks, or months of zero interesting things to say, I had a story. I've always found about a quarter of sexual gratification to be in the sharing of the sordid details – read into that what you will. *Look at me – sustaining life, washing shit-stains out of babygros and giving blowies.* Or at least, *a* blowie. So when I met up with some friends from school – some of whom had kids already – for coffee and cake the following week, I ventured a new topic yet to be discussed: who else is giving blowjobs in lieu of sex?

'You dirty cow!' one of them exclaimed, grinning at me and sloshing her cold tea over the muslin draped on her shoulder (see, everyone's doing it).

'NO WAY!' shouted another. 'God, I didn't even fancy a snog for about a year, let alone that!'

I glowed in their projections of me as a sexual dynamo. Until the third friend, usually shy and retiring, spoke up.

'Oh, I was shagging a week after giving birth. We had sex as soon as we could.'

This time all of us just stared at her, jaws hanging open.

'What, like actual sex? Actual penetrative? Penis in vagina?' I couldn't believe it. So soon?!

'Yeh! It was a bit uncomfortable at first, but it was mostly fine after a while.' She bent down to smell her baby's crotch for signs of shit.

I just couldn't imagine being touched like that. I didn't have one patch of skin that wanted warm hands to stroke it. In fact, I wondered if some of the nerve endings had been severed during labour because those familiar tingles and blissful shudders were a distant memory. Also, I couldn't yet sit down without first rearranging my bits. You know how a cat moves in circles on a cushion before sitting – padding around it, softening it up, making a little nest? I needed to do that, so that ideally there was minimal contact between the vagina and seat.

As I said, I was not on board with my new body, and never less so when faced with the prospect of sex. Before I got pregnant I'd class my sexual appetite as 'fair-to-middling', typical of most young professionals in a long-term relationship, but by no means voracious.

But now my body was so different, it felt like I'd be asking Rich to seduce an old lady with my face. And that just happens not to be the sexy fantasy it appears at first sight. Plus: *HI, MY VAGINA STILL HURTS, OK?*

I didn't feel sexual at all, and I didn't want to. I felt like a mother. My body was feeding, rocking, cleaning, wiping and cradling; my brain was monitoring sleep, appetite, bowel movements, nappies, cleanliness, routine, clothes size, cradle cap, rashes, feet, tummy time …' Suffice it to say, I wasn't sure I had the brain space to consider when and how the fucking would take place.

But when I got home that evening, I still put it to Rich that we should try sex.

'No, no, no, no,' he answered, 'You're not ready.'

I didn't like this. *I'LL tell you when I'm bloody ready*, I thought. I wondered why *he* was so quick to discount sex. Now, I'm not so gravely sleep-deprived and the hormonal surges have slowed to a gentle trickle, and I have a theory:

I'm sure you've heard that seeing your partner's vagina birthing a child is like watching your favourite pub burn down? Well, it's nothing like that. It's more like seeing your favourite vagina ripped to shreds by a rabid dog and then punched by a gloveless Mike Tyson, when he's wearing all his gold rings. Rich watched another woman taking a pair of scissors to my labia – that kinky atrocity didn't even make it into the *Saw* films and there's like eight of them.

At the time though, I was affronted. He'd always been a big fan of my vagina, what, now it was just discarded? *Sorry, is it not pretty enough for you, buster? Is it not all the more amazing for surviving near obliteration? DID IT NOT GIVE YOU YOUR FIRST BORN?!*

Another month passed, and Rich agreed: the bruises had disappeared. I was allowed to exercise (though of course, I didn't) and I started wearing normal knickers. Admittedly a thong still seemed a bridge too far, but the pants were definitely smaller and tighter than the initial post-partum bloomers. And I missed Rich. He was there all the time but he never gave me a friendly reach-around anymore, never so much as patted me on the bottom. I hated all that before, but now I was like, *TOUCH*

IT! Touch my ass! I missed the closeness. I wanted to feel a bit human and grown-up and lithe. I wanted in-jokes and illicitness. I'd moved so far away from being any kind of sex object, it was suddenly all I wanted.

Finally, Rich agreed it was time to try intercourse for the first time.

We approached the task with military planning. Of course the baby must be asleep and then moved, still in her Moses basket, from her spot by our bed to the cot in what would one day be her room. That in itself was a mission. Swing the basket, don't allow her to feel any motion of the transit at all. DON'T knock into the doorframe with what must be the widest goddamn Moses basket ever, and when you lower her down, use all the power left in your remaining half an abdominal muscle to do so smoothly, without a bump on landing.

Then we tested the monitor. Rich went into the nursery and made soft baby snoring noises, which I could hear perfectly clearly in the other room. Then I suggested he should come back to the bedroom and make sex noises so I could be sure the baby won't hear them if she wakes up. It would be good to gauge how loud is acceptable, just so we know. He didn't seem keen but I hissed at him 'It's essential,' and so he threw himself into the task, presumably thinking it might go some way to turning me on, ready for the sesh. It did not, as the baby woke up and stared up at me as her dad groaned and sighed like a showy prostitute in the next room. Rich and I agreed the moment had passed and reconvened the following night to try again.

Some perfunctory foreplay commenced on night two but we had forgotten how to do it. I smacked his hand away as he tried breasts first ('OUCH! For fuck's sake!! They're for the baby, not

YOU!'), then stomach ('Get off that, it feels like an empty bollock!') and finally, buttocks ('NO!'). He gritted his teeth and suggested I go on top and control the whole process. I clambered on, but it quickly turned out this was far worse. One breast – still encased in layers of nylon and soggy breast pads – sprung a leak, from God knows where, dripping warm milk into his eye. My stomach hung like a fleshy bum bag sweeping across his skin.

We switched back to missionary and agreed that this is basically like losing your virginity – just get on with it and save the pleasantries for next time. It was starting to feel like something out of *The Handmaid's Tale* – perhaps we would have to put a sheet between us, giving access to the vagina alone. He gingerly edged towards me. I was aware of something of chaise-longue proportions nudging what appeared to be my brand-new hymen.

'NOOOOOOOOOOOOO!'

And that's when I decided, sex just wasn't for me anymore. I would just abstain – simple. It's very uncomfortable, isn't it? And at best someone ejaculates, but what then? Another baby? Jesus, no. So the new plan was: no sex. Instead we were partners in this exhausting routine, high-fiving as we flopped into bed, always hopeful that this would be the night she sleeps through the night. Sleep became a commodity neither of us had any intention of passing up. Plus, a romance ban is easier to ignore when there's no clear bedtime, no downtime alone, and not much definition between night and day.

No sex for me. Kind of a relief, actually. I really needed to get on with kick-starting my social life with people who demanded no physical pleasure from me.

Where my mum friends at?

I honestly thought maternity leave is like a free holiday. *You have every day off, all the time in the world for your mates; it's like one big bank holiday! My social life is going to be bangin', wooooo!* But of course, the only way this is possible is if your social life has always revolved around the kind of drugs that make you incoherent and incontinent. Old friends were largely 'leaving us to it', assuming we'd be very busy with all the baby-rearing. The irony is, you actually have a LOT of time to socialise when you first have your baby. The trouble is, your hours don't suit other people's – as they're finishing work, you're winding down to the bedtime routine. They're ready for cocktail hour at 6pm, you're dangling your baby over a bath, hoping it doesn't shit on you. They're going out for supper, you're already asleep, storing up Zzzs before the 11pm dream feed when your friends will just be heading home to bed.

And if you *do* manage to schedule in a conversation, you'll only half-listen to what they say. Your sentences will be interrupted by explosive diarrhoea or a baby head-butting the table. And that's if you can remember what you were talking about for longer than 20 seconds.

My NCT friendships were lovely, but still embryonic. They were quite helpful at 3am when my baby was making a weird noise, but only if their baby was making the same noise. I thought the baby would serve as a hobby does in matching me up with other women. But here's the thing – you simply have the same schedules, give or take the odd nap. You don't necessarily have a single thing in common. Despite living in the same town and birthing in the same year, you might have seriously different approaches to parenting so you're not even on the same page about the one thing that you're expecting to bind you. All of that becomes obvious so quickly. Plus, you're asking to be liked for similarly sleep-deprived ramblings and acute vulnerabilities without any knowledge of what else there might be in you.

How could I be expected to make new bonds with people while delirious with tiredness and smelling of rancid cheese? And that was key to the identity crisis really taking hold, of course: no friends. Because without friends to pull you back down to yourself, your self-confusion can go from a minor irritation to total devastation. Even the few friends who I did manage to tempt down to see us every few weeks served to heighten my sense of confusion in many ways. I realised the full force of losing my sense of self as friends – old and new – held a mirror up to me and I found my image completely distorted. Whereas with Rich and our daughter, I was too tired to be anything but authentic – even if that was authentically falling apart at the seams – with my friends I tried out all kinds of hats in the hope that something would fit, that *I* would fit.

When normal people visit

One girlfriend came to visit me in those early weeks. I was sure I had to appear totally unchanged so she wouldn't run for the hills. I handed the baby over to her so I could gesture wildly throughout the full-length version of my birth story, swearing a lot, playing it for the laughs. I have a story, a great story! I was brave, I was strong, I pushed a baby out of my twat in less than 30 minutes!

'I didn't have ANY pain relief, nothing!'

Once the sting of the birth story was well established, I felt I had very little to offer in the way of chat. The adventure and certainly the drama sort of ended there to anyone not invested in the future of this miraculous kid. After three hours, my shell-shocked friend asked if someone else might want a hold of the baby so she could regain feeling in her arm. She'd bought the baby a tiny toy rabbit which I was convinced would choke her, so I acted all pleased, then stuffed it down the side of the sofa. *Why is she trying to kill my baby?* She eventually left and I realised I hadn't asked her a single question. I knew I had gone on about the baby too much, but couldn't think much beyond her yet.

My friend had come to see how I would navigate this new chapter. She was probably expecting some personal growth. Instead, in place of the friend she used to party with and confide in she'd found a little old nan. My friend – this beautiful, buzzing girl – had to sit quietly and listen to Nan repeat herself then lose her train of thought, sitting there in her armchair stinking of piss, oblivious that one nipple had strayed from under her ugly nylon bra. We had bonded over work, over filth, over fashion, over drinks, over the optimism of youth. Over our abhorrence of kids and the women who had them. And I officially had zip to offer on all those topics. But she was kind and returned regularly, never asking more of me than to tell her what this new life was like.

There was also a couple that visited us often, and treated us like rock stars. They too would ditch their sparkling social circle and rather than expect us to host and entertain, they'd bring us enough food for a week of buffets, and sit at our feet, asking questions with wide-eyed incredulity at the very feat of creating a child. They heaped praise on us and bigged up our achievement – keeping said child alive – as if it matched up to their brand-new business, which was already winning industry awards left, right and centre. They made us feel smart and accomplished, interesting even. The wife would sometimes drive down from London to just accompany me to the shops, to watch as I changed nappies and breastfed for the 95,076th hour in a row. Needless to say, these friendships endured and now we are through the other side, we even socialise in the ways we used to. Normality restored.

But still, our lives weren't compatible at that point in time, and with the best will in the world these visits couldn't be regular enough to keep me sane. I mean, was I really going to drag myself, my baby and the storage unit of paraphernalia I thought I needed to keep my child alive, to a nice quiet art gallery or even the local Côte Brasserie? (I did do that once and got the buggy stuck in that heavy velvet curtain they hang in the doorway – they nearly had to cut me out of the thing.) Would I spin round on the dance floors of Ibiza for a hen weekend, spraying out milk like a sprinkler? Nobody wants that. I'd most likely be absent for the big moments, and what would I be up for? What use would I be? I was a different friend, a bit of a shit friend, actually. I was unrecognisable. And they couldn't help me reclaim some of my old self because it wouldn't fit anymore anyway.

You just can't be there any more as a friend. I grew up with the prescriptive 'I'll Be There For You' blasting out of our tellies every Friday night at 9pm, and then from my CD walkman between 1995 and 1998, so I knew to be a friend you really had to *be there*. You have to drop everything in an emergency, or just turn up at their birthday parties no matter how much you've got going on. You have to at least ring them and check in. The way I'd been subsumed by the whole parenting thing meant I wasn't there anymore. I was coasting with the new friends to be honest, who understood we all kept weird hours now and could only accommodate emergencies that fit in with nap times. I was a rubbish friend and I lost the sense of agency in those relationships as my priority was singularly my kid's wellbeing. Nothing else mattered, which is of course a recipe for a disastrous social life.

Those friends can't always come with you to the 'mother side'. When you become a mum, a void forms between you and your old friends. It's inevitable. Even if your friends are already parents, because unless you're going through the whole process at the exact same time, there's still a gap between their experience and yours. Even if you can overcome your natural instinct to describe your first post-birth bowel movement in great detail to childless friends ('I held a sanitary pad over my bits, and it really helped me relax' is not winning chat, it turns out) and can keep your baby quiet enough to hold a normal conversation. Even if you strap that newborn to your body so your hands are still free to buy drinks and high five and light cigarettes like the old days. Even if your friend is happy to forget your past of partying, long brunches and late-night phone calls and will join you at every old National Trust house, to dash frantically around after a baby with a sadistic interest in prodding antique earthenware, leaving a trail of liquid shit in its wake. You're about to lose commonality, at least for a while. And as they slowly fall away, you realise how key they were to defining you, and how fragile your identity can become without them there to remind you.

The fannies that break together, stay together

Luckily, Lou got it. Our babies had arrived within four days of each other, and we were both tired and sore. Her friends were mostly in London too. We cried together, laughed while clutching at our fannies so nothing would prolapse and lamented over husbands, who could somehow sleep through anything.

But within a week or two, Lou had got really good at it all. She applied her sharp professional mind and management skills to the process and no matter how tired she was, she was so damned capable. She came to pick me up one day for a shopping trip to a neighbouring town and suggested she drive. But I had no idea how to take the car seat out of my car and put it into hers. I wrestled with it, with the baby sleeping inside it. I got sweatier as I knew Lou was on the approach, and I still hadn't managed to break the thing free of my battered Honda Jazz. When she pulled up in her massive new Audi, I was crying, my top half inside the car, my bottom outside in the rain. She told me to get in and watch her baby, while she swiftly clicked the buttons to release the car seat and slotted it into place in her own car. Effortlessly.

When I was with Lou, I *always* felt exposed, metaphorically speaking. I started so many sentences with 'I used to be …' to try and convince her I was a worthwhile person, whether the adjective was capable, glamorous, bright, adept or articulate. *I used to go on work trips all the time*, I wanted to tell her. *People trusted me to represent, I was good at my job, I was a bit like you.*

*But I've been totally subsumed by all this, and I don't understand
how you haven't!* I wanted to say the right things so badly so of
course I sounded insecure and thick. When did I become this
pathetic person? I needed her to know I'd seen things, I knew
people. I did some stuff, once. We didn't have the kind of history
old friends shared to help define one another in the hazier
moments. I was actually incredibly proud of how I was managing in private, but for some reason it all paled into insignificance
every time she had to fish my glasses out of the pram for me.

Lou was using the 2am feed to start looking for new nannies,
draft contracts, research nurseries. She was only having three
months off before re-joining the world of work with a new
promotion to get stuck into. She'd been promoted while on
maternity leave, for God's sake – that's how good she was. I was
re-watching the same episode of *Cold Feet* over and over again
because I kept nodding off and almost smothering my baby to
the tune of James Nesbitt's sexy groaning. God, Lou was brilliant. And usually I thrived around brilliant women. But instead
I felt puerile and slow.

One night, Lou and her husband invited us over for supper.
We were all finding it hard to work out how a night out would
look for us since it was too soon for babysitters and we were
stuck in the sticks. So the babies would sleep upstairs while we
had supper and danced the night away in their living room. *This
is where I show how fun I was, still am,* I thought. *Wait for it,
guys! This is my natural habitat!* But I couldn't do it. I was
exhausted and shaken. I couldn't comfortably arrange myself to
look relaxed and excited all at once, I was very aware of all my
body parts looking awkward. I was way too scared and highly-
strung to get drunk. I suspected the bottle feed – our first –

wouldn't go to plan, and knew of course I should have tried it out before, to make sure the baby would take it. I wouldn't tell Lou I hadn't planned for it properly.

Again I was thinking, *I wish Lou had been around in the old days, I used to love a drink.* The other three danced around, singing and laughing, while I sort of jogged on the spot, holding onto my boobs, which had started to ache. I wracked my brain for something to say and blurted out,

'So which day are you starting back at work, Lou?'

The mood was totally floored, needless to say, as she stopped dead in her tracks and told me it was the following week, welled up and swiped at errant tears.

Good one.

So Lou went back to work and I was suddenly completely friendless during the week: Mummy No Mates.

CHAPTER SEVEN

6–12 MONTHS

We are never going to socialise again. We are never going to have sex again. My vagina is never going to be the same again. WE ARE NEVER GOING TO SLEEP AGAIN.

After six months we just got used to the idea that life was going to be hell forever and we'd probably never sleep again. Sleep was still the most urgent of all our problems. We had tried everything. Nothing available via Amazon Prime had worked, no amount of white noise or super-soft muslin squares was going to sedate this little motherfucker, of that we were sure. But we'd moved up another babygro size and I moved down a cup size, so progress was being made.

As long as I was at home and NOBODY QUESTIONED ME, I could cope. *I don't need friends because actually, it's pretty exhausting to haul ass out of here and I might as well carry on sitting down.*

The really crazy thing is how happy I was, in spite of all the physical harm I felt I was experiencing. Her calls were the reason we were awake more than we were asleep and yet …

WELL, WOULD YOU LOOK AT THAT FACE! She quite cunningly became more responsive and giggly. She sat up like a tiny drunken uncle, waving her arms excitedly and then collapsing back in a pile of cushions, or better yet, face-planting the floor and laughing uncontrollably. She craned her neck to get a look at me if I moved from her eye line, hollering noises that could well have been 'Mamam' if I listened hard enough.

And when she did sleep – what an angel! I almost wanted to wake her again just to tell her how lush it was when she slept and how much I loved her. Of course I never did – that's the most fucking stupid thing I've ever heard. I quite aggressively pinned Rich to the sofa when he expressed the same thought, in fact.

And so, there were more moments of thinking how wonderful motherhood was than the other thought: that I'd sell the house and my car for the chance to sleep for longer than four hours. She and I were a little team. It felt like she liked me, despite my obvious desperation, and it was as if she wanted to thank me for the night feeds as she smiled endlessly and clapped for me, sensing perhaps I needed reassurance. She nestled her head into my neck for comfort, looking earnestly into my eyes and giving me one of those gummy smiles that makes you feel like you must be the smartest, most wonderful person in the world for them to look at you like that. Her little fists closing around my fingers or stroking my chest as she fed – it was all choreographed to undo all my cynicism and anger and selfishness. The warm weight of her, wrapped in a quilted sleeping bag was the most precious thing. I was falling harder and harder for her when I thought I was as much in love as it was possible to be – my capacity for love was just swelling every day, it was insane.

I suspect that's also why so many people experience marital problems around this time – there has to be someone to blame for the sleeplessness and moodswings, right?! And it's quite clearly not the kid. Cue a little marital discord, guys.

So, either Rich was a dick or I was a bit tired, overwhelmed and without an outlet for my dark side. It all manifested around a single subject – when would the baby be moved into her own room?

Rich's beef was that she could barely fit in the Moses basket anymore. I suspected he also thought he'd get laid more if there was no longer a mewling child in the room, always on the verge of waking and pointing at his naked butt. But moving her into her own room was something I'd been putting off – 1. Because I was an Earth Mother, of course, 2. Because I didn't fancy the commute to the nursery. But after a few rows about cot-death at six months I agreed. It was a shock because I'd basically been awake and welded to her for six months and hadn't had the break away needed to witness a change. Each night felt like an endless river of slow hours and yet here we were six months in and it felt like it had gone in a flash. I'd had meaningful relationships that had lasted half that time, I'd owned most of my shoes longer than her entire lifespan, despite a bunion-causing tight fit.

So one night we placed her in her cot when she'd finished feeding. I went to sit on my bed and made myself wait a full five minutes before I ran back in to see her. She'd rolled over onto her stomach. *Oops, can't do that baby – that's a major no-no!* I rolled her back lest she risk probable death (that was the NCT stance of the time – no sleeping on fronts – it's probably changed again by now). She slept on. I gave it another five minutes, only to find her once again on her front. I rolled her back about 25 times before Rich persuaded me to go to bed.

'She can hold her head up – the risk is gone, I think,' he assured me as we settled down to sleep.

I woke again and again, running in to find her alive but lying on her stomach. She wasn't stirring, wasn't crying out for a feed, and she didn't even wake when I rolled her again.

But then around 4am I realised – she's SLEEPING THROUGH THE NIGHT. *This is the night, and she's sleeping through it! Oh my GOD!* And it happened again the next night. And the next night, and four nights into this heavenly new status quo, we felt ready to announce: we had a Good Sleeper™. At last. I felt clever and fulfilled, like I had the secret to happiness. *OK, so I'm actually really good at this*, I decided as she managed a 7pm–7am snooze. So smug. I didn't even mind that this whole saga had proved Rich right.

I was still knackered by the day-to-day minutiae of parenting of course, but when you have a Good Sleeper™ you have some time in the evening to 'adult'. You can go back to your pre-baby sleep patterns, or perhaps even better ones since you're probably partying a lot less. Plus, the old feeding-to-sleep was working during the day, too – she'd nap regularly for around an hour at a time after each feed. EASY! I was tired but serene. I was very much in my Beyoncé, Queen of Mothers phase, like those pictures she did when double pregnant in 2017, all Madonna-and-child esque once more.

'I feel like I finally understand religion and epiphanies and glory-glory-hallelujah,' I told Rich one morning after a solid six-hour sleep. 'I feel like this might have been down to holy intervention, don't you?'

Of course, we were such TWATS! As if that was it! As if we were just destined to sleep well forever now that our baby had discovered she could roll onto her stomach! AS IF LIFE IS EVER THAT EASY!

Mums can be MEAN

I felt strong enough to have another crack at making some friends. I was a bit bored now I was no longer fixated on sleep, too. Lou was long since back at work and we only hung out at weekends, so I needed something, someone. To talk about the extinction of my sex life, how great my kid was at sleeping, that kind of thing. I wanted to belly laugh, even if my pelvic floor wasn't quite up to it yet. At first, I replaced friends with Netflix, obviously. My husband and I began talking about Frank Underwood and Piper Chapman as if they were real people. But eventually I knew I'd have to suck it up and make some new friends.

'What did you do, Mum?' I was back at their house for the fourth day in a row, mainly because the village shop had closed early so the owners, Malcolm and Lesley, weren't around for our usual 1pm chat.

'I was totally alone. Totally. Your dad would occasionally drag us to whichever theatre he was working at, where I'd sit backstage and take advice from mostly gay dressers and the odd elderly actress, but then we'd go home and it would just be you and me. I cried and cried, but nobody heard.'

'Fuck! Well, that's bleak. No friends, though? Who did you ring and chat to?'

'Dr Miriam Stoppard. A couple of times. I got her number through Dad's agent. I mean, we didn't meet, but she talked me through a couple of your fevers. Then she changed her number, I think.'

'I don't know what to doooo …' I moaned, as my mum basically ignored me and waggled her tongue at the baby.

'This isn't like you, Grace. You've always been very quick to make friends. I think you just need to approach people with babies. Just zero in on the ones with buggies and say hello. Be brazen.'

I felt anything but brazen at that moment. I didn't look, feel or sound like myself so it would surely be doubly difficult to persuade someone to befriend me. *But then,* I thought to myself, *my mum did it without social media, didn't she*? She didn't have filters and Photoshop and the worldwide internet. I was hooked up, so to speak, and quickly found out that where we lived, it all started at Rhyme Time at the library in town. It was free – bonus! – and it was packed. And it was at 2pm, which meant there was ample time to get dressed, eat something, feed a zillion times and even accommodate an unexpected, up-the-back shit explosion after the first attempt to leave the house.

I looked around the library's kids' room, quickly appraising mums. There were two very distinct clans – I assumed two sets of NCT friends – one big group with very tiny babies and one smaller one with babies bigger than mine. Elsewhere there was a pair of teenage Goths and a stay-at-home dad. I sidestepped this unlikely threesome because their kids looked about three, and toddlers still terrified me. So many teeth. I bravely pitched up to the group with slightly older babies. The woman to my right politely asked the standard entry-level questions – name and age of child seemed to suffice – and then turned back to her companions. They were already past breastfeeding, well into weaning and nursery, so I shrank back with nothing to offer. They were wearing activewear, for Christ's sake! I then had to sit through a full 30 minutes of songs without knowing a single word or action. It turns out Miss Muffet was *not* eating her cares away. I felt STUPID for not knowing the words to a NURSERY RHYME! Then 'The Grand Old Duke of York' requires you to lift your baby up and down in regular reps like some kind of HIIT class. It was bullshit. And my baby slept through the entire thing.

I then had to wait a full seven days for the next session. I'd already decided I would try the group with younger two–three-month-old babies, a mix of startled fawns, trying to navigate colic and cranial osteopathy and projectile vomiting. *Well, I could excel here,* I thought. *Because I have done six months now and I know pretty much everything.* But as I approached them, I felt like I was in the wrong year at school, gangly and awkward. *I know how to make friends, COME ON,* I thought. On my mum's advice, I got brazen.

'Who wants to pop over the road for a cuppa after "Wind The Bobbin Up"?!' I sound like a holiday rep trying to round up students for a drinking game, with my mad grin and over-rehearsed opener. Silence. There was an awkward sharing of glances between the five women, and finally the leader of the pack – Dr Judy (doctors are the ultimate mum friends because they can prescribe) piped up,

'Actually, we're going to Alice's for tea today …'

More silence as I waited for the invite.

And some more silence. BIG pause. I mean, huge. Like, bigger than Alice's vagina since she pushed out twins. Finally:

'… You could join us, I suppose.' Alice did not want me to join them for tea. But I was going to. *Sorry, Alice! Mama needs a bloody social circle!*

Obviously, it was awkward as fuck. These women had been meeting up for the past two months now – there were a lot of in-jokes and family packs of baby wipes being passed back and forth. *Who do you ask for one of those things?* I wondered as baby sick started to crust over on my shoulder.

'So … how's … the garden?' someone finally asked me, just as I was trying to sneak a fully-saturated breastpad out of my bra. She startled me, and the pad slipped from my hand and slapped down on the parquet flooring like a raw salmon steak. We both stared at it.

What the hell are you doing? FUCK! OK, just breathe, relax. No! No! Stop that! Stop doing that weird smile that makes your chin stick out. Relaaaaax. Think of something to say, think of something to say, ask a question …

Pre-Baby-Me – a social butterfly, a real talker – was going berserk inside my head while the current me remained totally silent but for the creak of the upcycled chair beneath me. Crafty Alice had apparently found the time to paint all her furniture in Farrow & Ball Ammonite, a twin attached to each tit. The Other Mother looked at me expectantly.

Just as this woman struggled to get a conversation started with me, I was struggling to answer. It turns out it's all one big struggle nowadays, socialising. I used to be the life and soul of the party.

I think I'm smiling. Am I smiling? I looked down at the car seat to see my daughter was still asleep. *Wake up, kid, for fuck's sake, wake UP!*

'Sorry, I missed that, what did you say?' I was stalling.

'I just asked, how's the garden? Last week at Rhyme Time I think you said your husband was laying some decking and you were hoping to paint it grey?'

Jesus fuck, I'm boring! Is that really what I made time to talk about? Time I could have spent with my eyes shut, imagining not having to wear a bra anymore. I would have disappeared to the loo for a moment to gather myself, but where do you put the baby if you go to the loo? Leave her with these potential sex traffickers? Or balance her on top of the cistern? There's nowhere to run, nowhere to hide. Nowhere to pee.

'The garden is good. I mean, it's the right size, you know? We haven't done it yet – the decking or the grey paint – but … we've just been so busy, you know?'

This isn't me, I wanted to tell her. But The Other Mother looked relieved so I can't have done too badly. I realised she has sensed a reprieve from this banal conversation is on the horizon, because I've been 'busy'. I wince. I know what's coming next. My least favourite question is on the tip of her tongue.

'Oh, what have you been up to?'

Feeding, changing, cleaning, feeding, burping, eating, eating, changing, eating, feeding, burping, cleaning, changing, bathing, trying to poo, crying, cooking, dozing, boxset watching, feeding, rocking, rocking, rocking, dozing.

'Oh! You know!' I don't know what I meant by this, and neither did she, but it doesn't matter because her baby woke up and she was busy. Thank Christ for that. I went back to my cold cup of tea, which tasted like flour. The cup had a picture of a chicken on it and brown rings inside like a tree. My lip caught on the chipped porcelain. I quickly licked away the blood so the mums wouldn't see and think I'm weird.

On paper I am somewhat of a mum-catch. I am a writer, I work in an enigmatic world of glamour and frivolities, I meet celebrities, I go to London, I travel abroad. I should have awesome anecdotes. But my brain is addled. 'Baby Brain', Judy called it and she's a doctor so I assume it's a thing. I couldn't remember yesterday or the day before, which day it is now, what we did last weekend. I flounder, hear the most boring things sliding out of my mouth but totally lack the dynamism to change tack. If I met me last year I'd have run a mile. In fact, Pre-Baby-Me would have run straight past this nightmarish room with its snot-encrusted muslins and browned Fisher-Price toys, ducking from view as she passed the window. I tried to tune in to the conversations going on around me, to pick up some technique tips. They were talking about a 'buggy babes' workout, mum tums, stroller recalls, nursery schools, the nanny who wouldn't stop looking at her phone … It was becoming a chore, trying to remember their names, their kids' names (all the kids look the same) and fielding their questions, all of which felt like a loaded gun: *have you brushed her teeth, brushed her gums, used a dummy, quit sugar, quit dairy, considered Montessori, tried Lanolin, moved her into her cot …?*

Was all this chat flowing so naturally because they'd been desperate to become mothers? Is that why I was struggling to fill in the gaps, because I wasn't ready for this? Were they just immersing themselves in this stuff because it's what they'd always wanted, what they ached to fill their brains with? Like when people get engaged and devote days to picking party favours and seat covers? Case in point – for my wedding I left everything until the week before and felt accomplished when I managed to pick up a veil from a fancy dress shop with just two days to go.

'I finally collected the Baby Bjorn bouncer yesterday, guys!' It's a mum in a Breton top and skinny jeans (standard issue mum uniform, topped off with a glittery ballet pump from Boden that screams, *I may be sensibly attired but I still have disco feet*) and she was positively glowing. I understood completely – I had heard it's like a babysitter has turned up in your living room with one of these things. 'Oh my God, it's the best, isn't it?'

'The best! He's just getting SO good at bouncing in it!'

'It's the best! Is it the best? Because we haven't got it yet. Everyone says it's the best. Is it really the best?'

'It really is, THE BEST!'

'Right, I'm just going to get it. I'm going today, I'm just going to get it. Online, obviously.'

'Obviously. Oh, you'll love it, it's the best.'

Pre-Baby Me tutted in my head, slipped a manicured hand inside her bag to fish out her phone and Tweeted something cutting. *I know, I know. But they're right, it is the best. And I'm desperate for adult company. I've lost all my old friends, I need new ones, damn it! You're actually being a bit bitchy. And I'm fine actually, fuck you very much, Pre-Baby-Me.*

Oh God, now Judy's sitting down next to me. What's her son's name … Jack? Jacob? Little Judy? Pre-Baby-Me rolled her eyes.

'Come on then, Sam, let's sit down here. Oh, Sammy-Sam! Oh, you're such a little bookworm, aren't you, darling? He absolutely LOVES his books, this one.'

That's not a fucking book, Judy. Pre-Baby-Me was at it again. *It's some fabric flaps with some stripes on it. There are no words. And he's chewing on it. He's probably ingesting a fair amount of cotton fibre, actually.*

'He so is, Judy! He just looks very wise, doesn't he? You can tell he's very bright.'

Judy treated us all like nurses. I put her buggy in the car boot for her and handed her Sam's soggy 'books' once she's strapped him into the car seat. I was not her friend, I was her assistant. And she was so competitive via the kids. Which was futile because they didn't really do much yet. So it was basically over how much formula they'd chugged or how many shits they'd done. She said things like, 'I won't have any of that nonsense, Sam,' and 'I can't WAIT to get back to work and use my brain!' *Jesus, my brain has never been worked this hard,* I thought. I didn't like who I was around these women. I'm sure they were perfectly nice, but there was still so much work to do to get to the point of being relaxed and open with them. It was exhausting and I was already knackered. I needed the common ground to be really obvious, I didn't have the energy to dig for it. I admitted defeat and promised myself an hour of *House of Cards* when I got home.

I took to sitting with Stay-At-Home Dad at Rhyme Time, listening to his lengthy list of parenting tips. I had quickly realised he was reciting Gina Ford but I couldn't face the others, and he expected very little in the way of replies. I hated Stay-At-Home Dad because his kid was always ill but he insisted on bringing him nonetheless. I have always had an issue with vomiting and catching bugs in general. Even the common cold can mean 1. You AND your baby AND your husband are ill,

2. Nobody sleeps for a week, 3. Having finally nailed sleeping through, you have to start all over again, 4. My mum won't come near because she has asthma, and so I can't offload the extra washing to her for up to a week. It's all very well being stoic and not encouraging a sick-note child (hi, I am that child) but it's as if there's no concern for the consequences. The missed holidays, nursery sessions, family parties, that narrow window your husband and you have booked in as the one opportunity for sex that month …

'Don't get too close,' they say with an eye-roll, 'Little Jacob was up all night puking!' As Jacob runs up to your child and licks her teeth.

As I ducked to avoid snotty kid's fifth hacking cough, which is basically acting as a catapult for a sinus system which behaves like Noel Edmonds' Gunge machine, I wondered if I could just rest my head here on the floor for a minute, I was so tired.

Then it happened. In she walked, a vision in a duffel coat and woolly hat, chubby six-month-old on her hip. I knew her! I'd had a holiday job at her sister's boutique during university, and had shared a couple of shifts with her. Marianne! She'd moved to London to be a designer at a glossy magazine, but now here she was in the same town as me again and wielding a baby as if it was a friend-magnet. I couldn't believe my luck and waited for a posse of NCT friends to follow in her wake. None followed.

'MARIANNE, MARIANNE!' I screamed. Everyone was alarmed and all the babies began to cry but this miraculous woman still sauntered over and after a moment of kind but confused smiles, thank God she recognised me. And just like that, I was A Friend again. Not only did we have a whole bunch of things in common from the pre-baby years, but our kids were born just a few weeks apart, we'd both landed in the countryside with a bump and were still reeling as exiles from Soho's magazine district. She hadn't bothered with NCT because her two best school friends had their babies just four months previous, but otherwise she hadn't met any new friends because of an awful round of mastitis, infections and blocked ducts. PERFECT! Of course I was sympathetic, and over-awed as she'd fed through the whole fiasco, even when she'd been hospitalised so they could drain pints of pus from one infected boob – but it meant she too was a social pariah. YAY! We saved each other, first with garbled verbal diarrhoea about all the shared joys and traumas, those glorious hours where you say everything and it just spills out of you, hour after hour, breathless rushes of information. Then in companionable silence, the best kind. She knew all the hottest clubs – Mumbabas singing group at the 12th Scout Hut, Acorns at the Baptist Church (they did give your kid a bible and sang hymns rather the nursery rhymes, but they also had the best tea) and Baby Sensory, which did cost a fair whack but there were no religious overtones. Thanks to the infected tits, Marianne was new to all this too, so we faced them together. We also spent a lot of time alone, outside, marvelling at mums with multiple kids at the park, dodging llamas at local farms. A goat once ate the piece of paper my baby was holding onto. It's savage out there. We actually felt more comfortable in skanky village halls once we'd realised all the cafes and restaurants got a bit snippy when our buggy brigade of two rocked up.

Sex and ~~The City~~ Vaginal Dilators

Another interesting development soon arose – Rich seemed to be after a shag. I was less mopey, less drippy. Sexy! Rich was sleeping more too. We were both rested. The baby was in her own room, it was just the two of us. We felt more like our old selves. Or rather, now there were no obvious obstacles, the lack of sexual intercourse was like the big blue-balled elephant in the room, so we tried again. But when we did try and get the penis into the vagina it was like trying to give birth in reverse, like he was trying to break me in two and set fire to my insides, or rather outsides since he couldn't make it past the entrance.

'Did it get bigger? Your dick is bigger!' I shrieked in horror, kicking his shoulders.

It was soon clear: the gate was sealed. The hymen was stronger this time, it was firm with renewed resilience.

I went to my gynaecologist to see if I still had a vagina. She investigated with what she said was the smallest speculum on offer. I cried and moaned, 'Owie!'

'Well, Grace, that is a designer vagina. Tight as a drum. They've stitched you up a little too neatly perhaps, but they haven't done a bad job at all.' She was admiring my vagina, which gave me a frisson of pride, obviously, but the fact remains, it wasn't fit for one of its designated purposes. I didn't want a designer vagina. Designer handbags might look good, but you're often hard-pushed to fit in more than a lipstick. I needed a bag-for-life, not some tiny clutch.

'The hormones you release when breastfeeding can play havoc with your libido, and if you *are* up for it, you'll most likely be too dry and your muscles won't soften in the same way,' my gynaecologist explained, proving her point with a transvaginal probe. 'It's very inhospitable. You need to stretch it out.'

I winced at the thought.

'We do prescribe vaginal dilators, but they're essentially ugly dildos. So I can do that or I can send you to Ann Summers and you can get something prettier. It's up to you. And you'll need a bucket-load of lube, obviously.'

'So, are breastfeeding and sex just mutually exclusive? Should I even bother with sex until I've finished feeding?' I must have looked stricken, because she gently slid the probe out of me, lube slopping down my bottom, and patted me on the knee as she handed me a paper towel.

When I got home, the in-laws had arrived. Perfect! I waited until *Corrie* was on and I was fairly sure they weren't listening to tell Rich: we might have to choose between sex and the continued nourishment of our kid.

'Well, six months of breastfeeding is great, bubs,' he said, mind made up, 'you shouldn't feel guilty about stopping now. High five!' I left him hanging, obvs. *How can I give up this thing that we're constantly told is benefiting her, just so YOU can get laid?* I change the subject: my vagina is now designer, by the way.

'Really?' he plainly did not agree. The man with one designer item – his wedding trousers from Hugo Boss (he didn't shell out for the jacket to make it an actual suit) – didn't deem my vagina worthy of the designer tag. 'If Chanel did really messy-looking patchwork false pockets made of raw wounds, I suppose.'

I did not feel comforted by this, and did not get excited about stretch-by-dildo. It was going to hurt and anyway, when would

I fit in this new regime? I was already having to milk myself, change breast pads three or four times a day and try desperately to conserve every remaining hair on my head – this seemed like yet another self-care necessity which would have no impact whatsoever on the way I look and so = pointless.

That said, I was hankering after a project, I did need a goal. All the NCT lot were finding new ways to make use of their maternity leave as the mortality of the kids became less precarious and they napped more. One was remodelling her house, another was thinking about starting her own business and a third was putting her house on the market. *My goal could be a wider vagina – why not?* I decided to ignore my gynaecologist's advice to start small with the tiniest of the Russian doll dildos and build up to penis-size and instead just go straight to actual penis. Using a penis would mean someone else benefits from the process and we could call it sex rather than 'dilation'. And if Rich could do Insanity three times a week, he could damned well put his back into making my vagina a more welcoming environment for penises. Luckily, I know all the right words to entice him.

'Come on, sexy, stretch me out! Haha! WAIT, NOT LIKE THAT, JESUS CHRIST THAT HURTS, YOU ASSHOLE! OH, I HATE YOU!'

He resents the telling-off when he's in the throes of passion. He gets a bit grouchy, actually.

'Well, do you want it or not?'

'ACTUALLY, RICH, THERE IS SOMETHING CLINICALLY WRONG WITH MY VAGINA! SO, I'M VERY SORRY IF IT'S A BIT TRICKY BUT … BUT … I'VE BEEN DIAGNOSED! I MIGHT NEED A VAGINAL DILATOR!'

Of course he couldn't stop laughing at this. I removed myself from under him and tutted.

'What is that, like a winch, or a crowbar of some kind? HAHAHAHA!'

'Pull yourself together, you dickhead, you're a FATHER!'

'No, no, wait! Is it like a picture of Ryan Gosling cuddling puppies?'

'WELL, IT WON'T BE SO BLOODY FUNNY WHEN MY CERVIX COLLAPSES AROUND YOUR COCK LIKE A VICE!'

Of course, when he had stopped laughing long enough, we had to work out when and how we could make sex a semi-regular thing. The space between our room and the nursery is three feet, so it had to be a silent event. She mostly slept for three-hour blocks before waking for a feed. Too close to feed time and my boobs would be jizzing out milk, too close to when she fell asleep feeding and I was drowsy and starving hungry. I would also need to have left a decent amount of time between eating and shagging so I didn't get a stitch (that's a real thing – it happens to me all the time).

Suffice it to say, there was no room for spontaneity, which is one of the key pillars of sexiness. Scheduling and preparing are boner killers and you can't just *tell* your fanny to get a-tingling. Without the desire for sex, you're totally reliant on foreplay. And since that hadn't been working out brilliantly for us either, we introduced other … elements. I would need to have about 20 minutes to organise the necessary tools to make penetration an option. This had become a combination of two types of lube and obviously a condom because I am not a complete idiot. It turned out my new vagina was also quite sensitive so we had got through five condom brands and four types of lube in pursuit of a non-burning sensation. Also, a vibrator was factored in on my gynaecologist's advice ('You need to give yourself a wide-on' – her actual words). But most vibrators are penis-shaped and sort of bash up against the actual penis, like a penis war. Or else it's so big it'll grind between your pubic bones in a most upsetting way.

On the occasions we got the timing right and our daughter didn't wake up we would creep into our bedroom and more often than not she'd sense something was afoot and start wailing, breaking the moment. Other interruptions included calls from my mother-in-law (who was able to sense exactly when her son was about to plough into me), a bleep calling Rich into work, and me issuing too many instructions. 'Not like that! Left a bit, slower, bit lower. No, no, stop dipping in and out like that! IT'S A VAGINA, NOT A BAG OF SHERBET, YOU TWAT!'

Rich has the patience of a saint, but also quite a large penis, so it was tough on us both. He persevered though, looking up sex-toy reviews in earnest to find the best possible aids. He became quite the connoisseur.

'Only one speed? Come on, Seven Creations!' he muttered under the blue-ish glow of his laptop. He eventually earned a loyalty card at one stockist in particular. I have a lot of GWP pocket rockets and free samples of lube.

I stopped calling my vagina 'fouff' around that time – it was far too dainty a name for something that had done battle with a child four times its size. It was simply called The Vagina, as if it was an add-on to me, my right-hand man, partner in crime. But far less sexy and French, of course.

I concluded that my sexual side had to be shelved. It's not like I was obsessed with sex beforehand, but it was definitely a part of who I was. Ever since I'd finally escaped my all-girls high school and become boy mad at college, I liked how men responded to me and the way they could make me feel. Two years in, I lost my virginity to my first proper boyfriend, and so experimented within a very safe relationship, earning my stripes in my parents' spare room over an 18-month, weekend-only spree. At university, I had a couple more boyfriends. I managed a few al fresco shags, and one on a bus that made me feel very experienced and worldly wise. I actually once won a prize for flirting, and my God, I had fun.

When I got together with Rich, it was like I'd reached the pinnacle of sexiness – I was 20 years old and so at the time both he and I thought I was the sexiest thing ever seen (IRL) and that felt amazing. Although I definitely wasn't on the market or flirting for Britain anymore, sex still ran through my humour, my writing and the way I dressed, to an extent. I no longer thought of myself as provocative in those skimpy clothes, but I liked the idea that I was expressing a young, sexy side with a few threads and sometimes tit-tape when the occasion called for it.

But even the clothes I considered slightly sexual and my modest collection of sheer underwear were shelved when I got pregnant. They seemed faintly ridiculous all of a sudden. Even pants and French knickers. So here was another swathe of my personality that was simply eliminated, not just from my sense of self – and wardrobe – but my relationship, too. *Still, the baby's sleeping through*, I concluded, *at least I'm not totally shit at everything*. Cue: things getting a little bit worse just to remove that sense of self-assurance …

Unsolicited advice is NEVER welcome

I was at a baby music group in a scout hut, keeping myself to myself, occasionally spilling my guts to the kindly lady who runs the groups but basically staring into space. The crack in the plastic chair I was slumped on kept snagging the skin of my thigh. This was everything I dreaded about motherhood, really, but my standard for things I enjoy doing had plummeted since drinking and staying up late were all forcibly removed from the table. Perhaps this wasn't so bad? In fact, as my baby jabbered away, arms waving enthusiastically as a lady with a maraca in one hand belted out various nursery tunes a cappella, I thought, *I am educating my child, tending to her sensorial needs and I don't even need to move. I am an amazing mother!* Pride always comes before a fall though, doesn't it? So this was probably the first little stumble, which would eventually develop into me face-planting the hard, jagged concrete of parenthood.

After 20 minutes of songs, the mums got up to make tea and pass round Custard Creams, and I settled back in my chair, deftly covering one shoulder with a large muslin cloth and tucking my baby beneath it to latch onto the already drippy boob. She suckled for all of five seconds then closed her eyes and was perfectly still, nipple resting on her lower lip, but most definitely asleep. I sighed a contented sigh. *Someone will probably bring me a cup of tea in a minute, maybe even a biscuit.* A portable heater was blowing warm air that only smelt *slightly* like dead rats right into my back. *This is the life,* I thought.

A mum I hadn't seen before sidled up to me and took the neighbouring chair.

'Are you feeding her to sleep?' she asked, smiling kindly.

'Oh yeh, it totally works!' I was smug mother of A Good Sleeper™.

'I'm a sleep expert, and the thing is, if she's used to being nursed to sleep, it might make it tricky down the line for her to go to sleep without it. You know, when you stop breastfeeding.'

'Sorry, you're a WHAT NOW?'

'A sleep expert. Nursing to sleep is never the answer.'

I looked down at my sleeping cherubic angel. *Have you SEEN my Beyoncé-serene face? Check out the other mums, they're tearing their hair out! I'm Beyoncé-serene, bitch! Tricky, is it? Fuck you!* Also, I felt sleep experts ought to announce themselves before they ask questions like, do you feed her to sleep? She should have had a badge or sandwich board in my opinion. Fancy sidling up like that, all anonymous. She stealth-advised me. Dropped a truth bomb on me, like a ninja with a Gro Clock.

'But … it works. She's A Good Sleeper™ … it … works, it works,' I stammered. Just then, the sleep ninja's charge climbed onto her lap. 'Naptime,' he said sleepily and laid his head on her expert shoulder.

'Got to go,' sleep ninja smiled again, warm and generous, presumably unaware she had given me The Fear. 'Ted always likes to nap at this time, and I'm sure you want to get your little one into her cot for a proper nap, too.'

'I surely will,' I shouted after her, following up with a loud 'It works' for good measure.

I was stumped. Wasn't I doing exactly what I'd been told to do by every healthcare professional, nay PERSON I had heard from since giving birth? I kind of thought – after the barrage of pressures from every camp – that breastfeeding was a good thing. I decided to ignore her, because this impending trickiness didn't sound likely. This wasn't the threat of cortisol surges and future mental health issues, it was just like a potential inconvenience and a few sleepless nights at some stage. Nothing I couldn't handle.

I naïvely thought a good sleeper was one who slept well. Actually, a Good Sleeper™ – I now know – is a baby who is laid in his cot awake but drowsy, who snuggles down unaided, smiles because he loves sleeping and knows it is good for him, and coaxes himself into a 12-hour sleep. He naps right on schedule during the day, sometimes three times and his mum does a spin class, redecorates the spare room and completes a PhD while he rests. I've read every book going and I'm still not sure HOW you get a good sleeper. What I was doing was drugging my baby to sleep with breast milk. If she roused, I shoved the boob back in before she had a chance to make the noise that woke us all properly, and within minutes she was asleep again. Life was peaceful, the night passed without a whimper. During the day if I had something to do, I could just sling out the boob and within seconds she would be napping, sometimes for up to three hours. I conducted many conversations, ate meals unimpeded, even managed to jump-start my writing career again.

I'd seen *Supernanny*, with the kids who wildly ran from room to room at bedtime, bouncing off the walls, eventually passing out on the 648th time their bedraggled parent popped them back in their beds. Kids that fought against sleep, their parents, the system, even the formidable Jo Frost, with every ounce of their being. I did not fancy that battle myself, but nor could I see our peaceful little angel becoming one of those fighters. Six months in and we'd only heard loud crying twice: once when someone sneezing had startled her and once when she'd rolled off the bed (I know, I know – it's OK, she was fine). She murmured when she had her jabs but didn't cry, she smiled all the time, even in her sleep. It wouldn't happen, I was sure of it. She's used to sleeping, that's the important thing, the habitual patterns. It's fine, it worked.

However, this phase would not last, of course, because my fall was overdue. I was soon to go from Beyoncé-serene to 2007-Britney, wielding an umbrella at rogue paparazzi who were trying to get a good shot of her freshly shorn head.

First, my breasts basically stopped working like they used to, as in she suddenly became immune to the sleeping pill effect my milk had on her.

The cherubic baby was angry with me, like a little junkie desperate for a fix, gripping my already bruised nipple and then jerking her head around. Niplash, I think they call it. Grinding her hard gums and gappy teeth around my nipple, pushing into my breast with her fingers, scratching in frustration. Obviously I remained silent so as not to break the calm we'd clung resolutely to, each night hoping this would be the secret to a peaceful sleep. But she wailed anyway, every night. Waking up every half an hour, a rage rising up from her belly and coming out of her gob in great gut-wrenching shrieks.

I resolutely stuck a boob in her face repeatedly until eventually she nodded off for a few moments, but like really forcing it in there like some kind of battering ram. *This doesn't feel so natural/glorious,* I thought to myself, *I can't see any Earth Mother forcing floppy nips into their offspring's mouth, using oneself as a human dummy, crouching over them on all fours. Why didn't we use an* actual *dummy?* I often wonder now. Because we'd been warned off them and didn't bother to investigate if the 1980s 'experts' (our parents) had based their dispiriting nonsense on an actual published paper or if they were just saying stuff for the sake of it. It's one of those obvious things we totally missed because OUR BRAINS WERE FUCKED.

Often she'd feed feverishly, thinking this was the answer, until she puked the excess milk all over her cot so that we'd be up even longer, changing, cleaning, wiping …

I'd created a reliance on having my boobs in her mouth and my arms around her to fall asleep, and now it wasn't so convenient for me to offer them, she was struggling to find a new way. I couldn't get her out of it. And then she was tired, and it was worse. This was nothing like the newborn days – this was a fresh hell. She was now a mobile 10-month-old, crawling tentatively from sofa to armchair and then careering about the house on two legs within weeks. She was fast because she had to be – the momentum was the only thing keeping her upright for a time – and we convinced ourselves that with all of this running around, she'd sleep better. She did not.

Then my husband placated me with the universal parental excuse: teething. 'It'll be over soon,' he reassured me – from the comfort of our bed, after a good eight-hour sleep, I might add – 'They just don't sleep when they're teething.' No new teeth appeared.

I cowed to her, not able to take the wailing and desperate for even a second of peaceful sleep. This entailed getting into the cot more than once – an interesting twist on co-sleeping – cramming my body into the small cage-like box and wrapping myself around her so she could chew on my nipples some more. I regularly lowered her into the cot still orally attached to me by the nipple, allowing my breast to stretch to unconscionable lengths. My nipples will always fold up inside a tight bra from now on.

I perfected the ninja-style retreat. I was like the Milk Tray Man – light step from cotside to the changing table, avoid the creaky floorboard; bend over the table, swing legs round to the end, being careful not to touch the floor; put one foot on the rug, grip the doorframe with both hands and swing out of the room to the safety of the hallway. Most likely the nipple was still in the baby's mouth at this point, but hey, the rest of me is outside the room. I curled up on the floor in the hallway, I slept hanging over the cot and I even found a five-minute nugget of peace with my head resting on the changing table, alongside the nappies. I was quite scared of her, actually, because the cortisol screaming stuff was happening even though I was being the calm baby whisperer or whatever such bollocks I thought I was supposed to be, and I felt out of control for the first time since my labia had been ripped open.

And the baby went from being my cherubic angel born without sin to THE LITTLE CRETIN, WHY WON'T SHE SLEEP?!

One night, Rich appeared in the doorway at about 3am when I had somehow managed to sleep through a particularly loud scream, even though I was standing up, and we began a row conducted in whispered hisses.

'WE NEED A PLAN AND WE NEED TO STICK TO IT!' He hissed, as I bent over the cot with both tits out.

I still refused sleep training as a viable option because the crying was threatening to crack my skull. So I started to scrabble around for an alternative. I read several books and established she was going through a 'Wonder Week' or a 'Leap' or some kind of existential crisis, but nowhere did I find an actual solution. The No Cry solution involved weeks of baby steps – sit next to the cot for a week, in the middle of the room for another week, then by the door, then in the doorway, then outside and so on, until finally you will be almost in your own room and hopefully they will be asleep. But I'd never make it past day 2, when she would look like she was suicidal and I'd be climbing back into the cot to reassure her.

Even though each evening we had a plan, based on various books, when it came to the delirium of 3am, those words had fallen out of our brains. It's easy to agree at 4pm that tonight you'll remain consistent, only pat her back once, stay within sight but not touching her. Yep, that's a good idea – it's clear and concise and we know how to do that. But when the kid is wailing and you're groggy you start to think perhaps this *is* cruel, she doesn't seem to like it, oh God, here comes the cortisol. Rich was still on the previous chapter – be consistent, be strong – but I was skipping ahead to a new phase where we ignore all advice and do what feels right. We couldn't make the books work – I needed the authors of those books to come in and do it for us. The instructions had stopped making sense, like when you say something too many times in a row and it sounds ridiculous. We were caught between the 'gentlest' who proclaimed sleep training a tragic and harsh sentence with dire consequences and the 'realists' who assured us it was the only thing that would work. So Rich would head in when I snapped that he wasn't helping, only to be shooed out again seconds later when I would bowl in and criticise whatever he'd decided to do.

I hated myself, I was scared Rich was going to tell me I was doing it wrong, and I was sick with worrying every evening as bedtime approached. I didn't know what the hell to do. And having crowed about how easy this parenting game was, I suddenly felt totally powerless and like a true failure. It didn't help that I loved her to distraction – I would never have put up with this behaviour from Rich! This kind of mental torture. But the love just dragged me further down.

Me: *I need sleep! I can't keep going in to stick my tit in her mouth, I can't!*

Books: *But your baby needs you. She needs your milk and your comforting arms. She has nothing without you.*

Me: *But I can't! I can barely lift her!*

Books: *WELL THEN SHE'LL DIE, MWAH HAHAHA!!!*

I was feverish, the thought of sinking into fresh bed sheets was almost sexual. I fantasised about sleep, it made my skin tingle to imagine my eyes closing. I thought everyone else was getting it. I hated my mum for telling me she was a bit tired because she'd been watching *EastEnders* on catch up until 11pm. I hated the postman for knocking on the door and waking my baby up. I hated myself for being such a shit mum.

It didn't help that I craved the two chemicals guaranteed to make my tiredness worse: caffeine and alcohol. I think the popularity of Prosecco and Flat Whites has risen at a similar rate, and perhaps in sync with the proliferation of confusing parenting books. The idea is that you book-end your really shit sleep with two chemical treats which do fuck all to improve matters but might make you feel buzzed for approximately three minutes.

At some point, that last feed of the day was enough to send her off to sleep again. I half-heartedly tried to 'put her down drowsy', but basically, feeding her to sleep worked again and I was half the woman I'd been before. Yeh, we didn't do anything special, it just seemed like the hellish bit was over and some kind of order had been restored. Our next plan was to nail nap times, because, we thought, *if she can go to sleep during the day without the boob, she'll get used to the idea of doing it at night and perhaps one will just segue into the other*. I was told that the more sleep they get, the more they want and need. Get them into a routine of napping and they'll come to expect sleep, to welcome it. Nap time became an obsession.

It was such a burning concern that my routine went like this: get up at 7am as she wakes and breastfeed for 20 minutes. Feed her breakfast and as soon as she's finished, whisk her back upstairs, change her nappy and hold her in the cot until she submits and falls asleep. Get her up after 45 minutes to an hour, and play with her, but if she shows signs of sleepiness – yawns, eye rubs, grizzling – whisk her back up to bed again for nap number two. Otherwise, feed her lunch and get her up to bed straight afterwards for that nap. Get her up again, play, and back for another nap, this time in the buggy, come rain or shine. Then up for a moment, feed her tea, bathe her and back to bed for good. A lengthy breastfeeding session, followed by up to three hours of placing her in her cot and offering reassurance at two-minute intervals.

I couldn't go out, I couldn't do anything, I was exhausted. I was spending at least eight of the 12 hours she was awake trying to get her to go to sleep. Rich once suggested we go out for lunch to just get away from it all for a bit and I had to explain to him, a social life was not my priority anymore and it was a completely ridiculous suggestion. IF SHE DOESN'T NAP NOW, SHE

WON'T SLEEP TONIGHT AND THEN I WILL KILL YOU! Long gone was the laid-back, 'she won't change us!' idiot I'd been just six months ago. I was a slave to the nap-time routine.

The advice was mixed though. 'Don't nap too close to bedtime otherwise they won't be tired enough. And don't let them nap in the car because it'll mess up their spines and you'll also become reliant on the car for them to fall asleep. But bear in mind that if they're reliant on being in their cot at home, you'll have to be home certain hours of the day every day and won't be able to travel far afield. Offer lots of comfort and support but not so much that she can't sleep on her own without you,' … and so on.

'DON'T YOU GO TO SLEEP NOW!' I was singing this loudly, so it wasn't as threatening as it looks on the page. But it was sung with the same sense of urgency and fear it implies. 'IT'S TOO LATE, STAY AWAAAAAAAAKE!' I was hurtling down the road to our house at 4pm, and having not napped once through the day, the baby's head was lolling and her eyes were rolling. I wound down all the windows until it looked like she was in a wind tunnel and sang loudly to her for the remaining 800 yards, throwing rice cakes at her. I jumped out of the car, ran round to her door, only to find her fast asleep.

The worst thing, other than the mind-numbing tiredness, of course, was the guilt. *Why can't I selflessly put her first anymore?* I often wonder. *Why can't I comfort her patiently and endlessly, why must I get so cross? Why can't my body cope? Why can't I do all that and not go mad?* Occasionally I thought it would be kind of brilliant to move Rich out of the bedroom so she and I could share. I could just roll over to pat her on the back and we'd go to sleep giggling, wake up cuddling. She'd never say things like,

'I'm lonely!' or worry about monsters sitting under her bed. It would be so much easier. *You'll be wishing those midnight cuddles back when she's a teenager who sleeps until noon*, they tell you. *I fucking won't*, I think. I'll still be tired so I'll just climb in with her. Also: making us panic about the fleeting nature of this baby bubble is NOT helpful, memes, OK?

PART III

THE CRISIS

CHAPTER EIGHT

CRISIS TALKS

I think I'm fine now. I mean, not FINE, obviously. Just OK. But it's fine.

Nothing huge happened. It was just a normal day. But a little spark – imperceptible to the human eye – was ignited, and that little spark would be the catalyst for a crisis. Soon I would fully realise that the me-that-was had permanently vacated the building and someone else had skulked in to replace her. Who? I don't know. Some bird.

It had been 10 months since my now walking-talking (well, almost talking – more like shouting random sounds that sounded a *bit* like words you knew) daughter came into the world. I was innocently chopping carrots for a lunchtime stew with one hand and pouring air-tea from a plastic teapot into my daughter's open mouth with the other when my phone rang. I looked at it in surprise – my mates didn't usually call, either because I'd ignored their calls one too many times as they clashed with bedtime/feedtime/nappy time, or because 'they didn't want to disturb' (or listen to another rant over the fact that there was zero relief available for a constipated baby). It was an old friend from school calling to say she was coming down in a couple of weeks.

'I wondered if you'd be around for a visit, but then I realised it's your birthday, isn't it?! So I'm guessing you already have plans?'

Shit. Yes. My 30th birthday was looming.

'Um … no plans as such. Why, what do you want to do?'

'It's YOUR birthday, dickhead! Spa day? Shopping trip? Cinema? Party? Come on, it's your 30th! You've got to do something! I don't know, what do you like doing?'

I considered this. *What do I like doing? Sleeping? Hardly a group activity. Do I like spas? I could sleep at a spa …* It reminded me of a French class when I was 14. We were practising for our oral GCSE exam and the teacher had asked, 'Qu'est-ce que tu aimes faire le week-end?' – what do you like to do at the weekend? It had to be something I could say in French, but I was basically too old for hobbies and too young to actually do anything I fancied doing independently, so I answered, 'J'aime aller a la discothèque,' and all the mean girls in the back pissed themselves laughing at me and I nearly DIED.

Put on the spot like this I couldn't come up with a single thing that I could be arsed to do. *Go to London? Oh no, so many terrorists. Go to the beach? UGH, sand, UV rays, water, sand. OK, do I like shopping trips? The cinema?* Surely going to the cinema was just watching a different TV while a babysitter watched yours? If I went clubbing, would I dance, would I drink? Could I do either of those two things? Plus, I had no money to spunk on non-baby items.

In the past, I'd been quite demanding of birthdays. I didn't let a single one pass without a party. Dance floors, holidays, parties, theme parks … But here was this huge opportunity for a big blow-out (if people felt duty-bound to attend birthday parties, that obligation is doubled when it comes to the big birthdays like 30ths) and I couldn't think of what would be worth the sizeable effort everything seemed to involve these days.

I felt like all the fun had been wrung out of me, like that part of my brain was switched off somewhere between giving birth and the 200 hours I'd spent in draughty village halls avoiding snotty toddlers. I mean, don't get me wrong, in those days if you'd propped me up in Bill's with a mocha and a sleeping toddler strapped into a buggy, I was a riot. If they'd got a lift, even better. But I was there so often the staff brought me my coffee without asking and a stack of napkins to stuff in my bra. It couldn't constitute a birthday treat.

Imagine: 'What did you do for your 30th?'

'Oh, I had an extra coffee, because I AM CRAZY!'

What *did* I like doing? And where did it all go, all that fun stuff that used to fill my brain?

Rich and I had sort of stopped socialising together by then. After a strong start of dining out, we'd become too tired and tied to routine to manage for long, and so to date our social life had been daylight hours only – Sunday lunches at the pub, NCT coffee dates, play dates, baby groups … I'd missed weddings and birthday parties, and Rich had been to countless occasions on his own. He was so cool about it (errr, opportunity to socialise and NOT talk about breast pads, YEH, ALRIGHT THEN!), but I knew it wasn't how he wanted to do things – basically single.

I liked picking our baby up at the end of a nap, her sweaty little head resting on my shoulder as I quietly sang to her. I liked the delight she took in slapping my tummy and watching it ripple, or in feeding her dolls. I liked the fresh-clean feeling of a new nappy, the gurgling smiles. The triumphant stagger from sofa to armchair and the wet, open-mouthed kisses with a fist in either ear. Keeping her nursery tidy, her nappy bag stocked, getting out stains, cooking something she'd eat. I liked watching her study Rich's kind face. I liked it when everyone else was asleep and I could watch something shit on TV. I liked the way she moved when Beyoncé was playing, the way she smiled like a lovesick teenager when my dad walked in the room. I liked it when she reached out her arms to me.

It occurred to me then, as I absent-mindedly stirred the carrots in a vat of water without switching the hob on, that I – the old me that liked fun stuff – was lost in being a mum. *I am permanently tired. I am mostly friendless. I am 100 per cent sexless. I only get excited when our routine goes to plan or over a 45-minute lie-in. I'm one-dimensional.*

I knew my 30th would warrant some kind of occasion – everyone would expect it and by ignoring it, I would be consolidating this persona as a washed-up, wrung-out has-been. But at the same time I was realising that the things I *did* enjoy in no way would count as a celebration. Because they were the solitary moments with my baby.

I started to realise the brutal struggle to maintain a corner of me ended when she was born. I didn't keep a lot for myself. *Has anyone noticed I've gone and there's a me-shaped mum in the space I used to take up?* I realised that I felt harmed by the whole experience, but was so confused because something that had given me unparalleled joy, meeting the love of my life, could have a negative effect. *I must be even more selfish than I'd thought. Motherhood IS supposed to be about self-sacrifice, isn't it?*

I was way too ashamed to voice these feelings – I could've gone to my mum but she was embracing grandmotherhood possibly even more than motherhood, and I didn't want to admit it to someone who was this invested in the child. I couldn't tell Rich because I still wanted him to think I was doing a good job, that I enjoyed selflessly devoting myself to our child, thinking it made him love me more. I didn't want to change anything or go anywhere yet. But I also started to worry that pretty soon everyone would realise I was no fun anymore. Rich would leave me as soon as the kid was all grown up, at this rate. So all I could do was agree to a birthday-by-numbers: a party with food and drink and dressing up.

Going out was the common facet of our otherwise wildly different personalities that initially fused Rich and I together as a couple. In our first year of going out we rarely saw each other outside of a nightclub, student union or a bedroom. Others bond over a love of books or a shared political belief system, Rich and I both loved getting trollied and showing off. The recipe was simple: a bottle of cheap wine on an empty stomach (obviously), anywhere between seven and 10 VK Apples in the club, shots to muddle, a pint of something murky and a pizza or battered sausage to round off the night. We were sexy, vivacious, fun and HILARIOUS.

He'd overlooked my mood swings and neurotic streak because I was a laugh and could hold my drink. I ignored the way he ate really slowly and his penchant for 90s rock because he wasn't afraid to look stupid on the dance floor. All very healthy, fruitful things to base a relationship on. I mean, we were like the country mouse and the town mouse, from opposite ends of the UK and totally disparate backgrounds, but then someone remixed the *Baywatch* theme tune and we were away. Obviously we had a bunch of other things in common (*The Sopranos*, *Peep Show*, *Anchorman*) but it might be nice to revisit this thing that was all about being young and carefree and fun. Perhaps it wasn't something we could afford to shelve just because we were supposed to have outgrown it.

Rich agreed a party was just what we needed and my 30th was the perfect way to make people feel like they *HAD* to make the long journey down to our cottage to celebrate with us.

NOTHING to wear

As we started inviting people – some of whom I hadn't seen since the baby had been around – I started to think afresh about what I looked like. Did I look like a mum now? There was the drawn complexion I'd feared, the trussed-up breasts, the neglected hair with three inches of regrowth.

And what would I wear? I wasn't sure what occasion dressing would look like now I was a mum. *What did I used to wear?* I wondered as I stood in front of my wardrobe, overwhelmed by the swathes of oversized shirts. I had once been fashion coordinator at *Vogue*, I used to get paid to put things together, pull out winning items to put on the pages of a style bible. Now I couldn't so much as coordinate the letters to SPELL fashion. It's tough for a seasoned clotheshorse to watch every thread stretch to snapping point and then be relegated, a part of a former life. The leggings and massive tops had become like a disguise, a stock uniform while decisions about what to wear were beyond me. I'd gone from thinking, *What will show off my boobs/bum/legs/*

collarbone to *What will cover up my arse crack when I bend down to retrieve a dropped sippy-cup? What can we NOT see my lopsided fanny through? What will keep my nipples covered but also allow them to be easily accessed in an emergency? What doesn't have baby sick or snot on it?*

I remember watching the Kardashians packing up Bruce Jenner's wardrobe when he became Caitlyn Jenner and she clearly didn't want the polo shirts and tracksuits of her former life. Clothes can be so indicative of who you are at any one moment, who you *were* in each phase of your life. And not only had my body changed, but the way I spent my time and would most likely continue to do so for at least a year had changed completely. I had used clothes as sartorial messages all my life – to establish an identity, to grow out of childhood, to attract boys, and as I grew up, to be taken seriously or to make me feel good. Or to conceal my throbbing imposter syndrome at any stage of life. I didn't know what I wanted my clothes to say anymore.

I usually shed the bulk of my wardrobe when I move house or just leave a phase behind, but I keep relics of those days each time. So my wardrobe was basically made up of short skirts from university (*maybe I'll wear them with tights and boots one day, or will need them for a Steps-themed fancy dress party,* I reasoned); poly-blend tops from my Sienna Miller boho moment circa 2004 when I had no tits and no money; two boxy LK Bennett skirt suits I'd bought for my first job at *The Times* before realising everyone wore skinny jeans and ballet flats; skinny jeans and ballet flats, and then a bunch of ill-fitting but expensive designer items I'd bought at sample sales when I worked in magazines, that mostly didn't fit but were discounted to the point of confusing me into buying them. This 'collection' included a Chanel tennis skirt, a too-tight black cocktail dress and a sheer bra-let. Since having the baby my mum kept dropping off her cast-off sweatshirts and harem pants, with the words, 'Thought these would be good for you know, just slobbing about.' At Christmas she'd even invested in four pairs of Abercrombie & Fitch tracksuit bottoms because I was apparently 19 again and lived in a Frat house. But otherwise I hadn't bought many new clothes since having a baby because I was still under the impression my body was in flux – *This isn't what I'll ultimately end up with, so why buy things that won't fit in a matter of months?* was my ethos. Yes, even though it had been nearly a year, I still thought everything must be temporary.

It was time for a rethink – the bodily changes had slowed right down, I no longer needed a top that unleashes boobs at any given hour. *Some new clothes might help me feel more like my old self,* I thought, cautiously edging the cursor towards the WOMEN section on the ASOS website.

I ended up buying a lot of slogan tees. Up until this point I hated them. Things like 'I'M TOO GOOD FOR YOU!' in lurid pink makes me squirm. But when you can't talk without sounding like a lobotomised monkey, you need clothes to speak for you. I basically wanted a T-shirt that says:

'I am so fucking tired I can't speak but if I could, I'd say something awesome.' But I settled for 'OH LA LA!' and 'ENFANT TERRIBLE', thinking myself witty and quite edgy.

I bought some skinny jeans and found I could basically fold my stomach up into them. I steered clear of spaghetti straps (I need a bra) and silk (a dribble and snot magnet), but found a nice selection of cosy cardigans … *NO! WAIT! STOP! NO*

CARDIGANS! CARDIGANS ARE FOR MUMS! I bought a neat leather jacket instead. Which, happily, would also wipe clean.

But what would I wear to a party? Not skinny jeans because I had cystitis AGAIN (stretching out the fanny was not without its problems). I decided my legs basically looked the same, so I'd get a spray tan and wear something short but capacious.

The spray tan

Back in the day I would rarely leave the house without applying a good coating of Rimmel Sun Shimmer. In fact, I often wore it in lieu of actual clothes. Once I left university that orange look fell out of favour, but I would get a spray tan for holidays, big parties and weddings. I have never tanned naturally – I go straight to red in five minutes flat, and working in beauty, I was schooled in both the threats of skin cancer and a leathery-hide complexion. I quite often got freebies with work so it became an occasional habit. It was like a pair of tights but less likely to ladder. I thought a spray tan might be just the thing to get me feeling more like that carefree, party girl.

I wasn't thrilled at the idea of getting stark-bollock naked, but I told myself: it's just a body. Nothing they haven't seen before. So there I am, bravely bearing my entire body – stretch marks, wobbly stomach, engorged breasts – standing in a sort of half-tent while the therapist busied herself next door. I pondered how to stand – hold my breasts? Hold my stomach? When she eventually came in, I was bending over to try and pull a toe-hair out, so that was nice.

She got started, directing me to assume the positions of the spray tan – it was the closest I'd get to yoga that year – and I clenched my teeth as the freezing-cold fluid was shot at my sensitised skin. She stood back for a moment to admire her handy work.

'What's this?' she asked, edging closer to my thighs. *Oh God, have I prolapsed,* I wondered, *or is there a massive crop of hairs I failed to reach with the razor?*

'You haven't had a little … accident, have you? Only it looks like something's … dripping.'

I looked down and saw the skinny white streaks striping my legs, little rivers coursing through the tan.

'I'm pretty sure I haven't peed, if that's what you mean. Maybe there's a leak in your ceiling?'

As she looked up, I looked down and located the leak. My right tit was dribbling. It had been dripping down my legs and now it was full-on spritzing. I grabbed both boobs and ducked down – no idea why, possibly so I didn't get her in the eye – explaining I was in the process of lactating. I hadn't thought it through – once again, tiredness addles the brain, OK? And if I *had* managed to get my tits spray-tanned with the rest of me, what would have happened when I went to breastfeed a couple of hours later? Would the baby have looked good with a dank-brown beard and moustache? Most likely not.

The therapist handed me a couple of cotton pads to place over my nipples and left me to get dressed. In my slogan tee that read 'CRÈME OF THE CROP'. Appropriate.

The party

On the morning of the party I busied myself around our garden, putting flowers in vases, hanging storm lanterns in the trees, kicking cat shit off the decking. I put our baby in a little party dress and ended up with five minutes to shower, do my hair and put on make-up. I spent three of those staring at her – she tugged at my wet hair, smiling.

'Hair? Hair. Hair,' she murmured as she gently put her fingers between the strands. In her eyes I was beautiful and just what I should be. I made all the right noises and had the right instincts of what to do next. I could slouch or lie down, I could make her laugh and knew when she needed a drink or something to eat. She made me feel like I was still OK. I wanted to stay here with her and her unerring approval, and not venture outside, where I'd have to consciously think about where to place myself and how to talk. Shit, when did this get so hard? My mum came upstairs to tell me to get a move on, and took the baby so I could get dressed and dry my hair. I had a little cry, sitting on the bed in my jersey nursing bra and massive knickers. I felt sort of shy and anxious and not at all like socialising.

COME ON, YOU WIMP! says pre-baby-me. PULL YOURSELF TOGETHER! GET YOUR SLAP ON! DRY THAT NEST YOU CALL HAIR! PUT ON SOME BLOODY HOT PANTS AND GET OUT THERE. THIS IS A PARTY, WE LIKE PARTIES!

I do it all, and put on a weird outfit – denim shorts with a very old Ghost top with a plunging neckline and a pair of espadrilles (I think, *I'll look like a knob in heels in my own garden*) and I got out there and started greeting guests.

I watched Rich telling stories, topping up drinks, laughing with our friends. He hadn't changed. I mean, he looked the same, and he still slotted straight in with everyone. He could talk about work, show an interest in their lives without glazing over … I realised that other than worrying about what he'll think when I feel I'm doing a crap job, I hadn't considered his feelings much. I tried to ensure he slept now and again, but I didn't think about whether he was enjoying this new life. He seemed fine, ever the warm host. *Lucky bastard*.

When you're at your lowest ebb, your self-esteem is at rock bottom and you're questioning every decision before, during and after you've made it, that's when the people around you will pick their moments to moonlight as your own personal judging panel. Unsolicited advice is the Donald Trump of the parenting world. In that, you thought everyone would know it's a terrible idea and then the majority stun you by doing it anyway. A lot of our guests had never seen us with a baby, so it was bound to happen. And what better place to start dismantling your confidence than at your 30th birthday party, a party where the only jelly is the post-partum mound caught up in your Spanx? Anyway, it turned out the party banter around me had declined as quickly as mine, with choice comments including, 'Give her some condensed milk to bulk her up a bit. She's quite small, isn't she?'; 'But babies look sweet with a tan!'; 'Don't give her formula, it stretches their little tummies'; 'You're STILL breastfeeding?!'; 'Daddy's looking really tired, I think it's time Mummy started a proper feeding routine now so the baby will stop waking him up in the night'.

What is clear about this feedback is that it's mostly in defence of their own decisions. Every choice you've made is seen as a comment on how they did it or if they're yet to parent, the bits that scare them. Also, they're outside of the fog so they can see in. They can see you wheeling around in circles and have what they consider to be the way out. But that day I was vulnerable and receptive, soaking it all up like a sponge in a bowl of piss. The absolute worst is when they talk to you through your baby. It's the ultimate passive-aggressive move. 'Oh, poor little thing, has Mummy not given you enough milk? Mummy needs to feed you more often, doesn't she, Poppet? Because you're just not growing very quickly, are you?'

I had a bit of a chat with everyone though and tried my best to filter the baby-related information. My excellent repertoire of fart noises and impressions of Mr Tumble – my number one skill when it comes to entertaining my 10-month-old – needed to be kept to the nursery, I know, but it doesn't mean they disappear altogether now I'm around adults. I kept looking for the kid – her cry called me back like a siren every so often, and at other times I caught glimpses of her with my mum and bouncing on the knees of friends. She was not looking for me, she was having a lovely time. I almost felt normal. At two o'clock I merrily stalked up and down the garden with Lou and our buggies to get the kids to nap in the shade. Everyone sang 'Happy Birthday' and I sat down to listen to a group of girlfriends discussing their love lives. I felt on the fringe of things but happily so. *This is quite fun*, I eventually decide.

Rich did the bedtime routine and I sneaked up just for the goodnight feed, which I lingered on, having barely seen her all day. She was content and asleep early, and I realised I have a garden full of friends, ample Prosecco and the night was young.

I could have a drink, it would be like the old days! It got dark and by candlelight we did some fairly sad dancing with an iPhone stuffed in a pint glass. Three Proseccos in and I was buzzing! Laughing loudly, sparkling, most likely dazzling everyone with my moves and witty remarks. An old friend I hadn't seen in years sidled up and attempted a high-five, which missed and bounced off my still slightly tingly tit.

'You've still got it, haven't you?' he said, giving me the thumbs up as he body-popped towards the shed.

I mused on this – interestingly not on the fact it was an unequivocally vile thing to say – but *yes, I bloody do still got it!* I think I was actually pleased to be objectified because I had assumed that wouldn't happen anymore. *Look at me, I am dancing and drinking! Look at my legs, they're out! Look at us go – baby's asleep, we're with the same friends, we're writhing around with style and grace. They're not bored, I'm not bored! This is my best life. Maybe we are unchanged after all!*

At 11pm I heard the baby grizzling on the monitor so I went up to pat her on the back. She quickly settled back down, I wandered into my room and my head began to spin. I vomited on the rug, then got into bed.

Three glasses of Prosecco and I was out for the count. What?! If this had been six years ago I would have assumed my drink had been spiked and protested to everyone.

Rich eventually came up to check on us and pronounced the party over, and the guests apparently filed out, wondering where I'd disappeared to.

I woke up the next morning with the worst hangover and drinker's regret, exacerbated by the fact that I had to skip our morning feed and spend all day chugging water so I'd be fit for the bedtime one. She didn't seem to mind, but obviously I felt like the lowest of the low. I hated the party and my friends and the Prosecco.

I dragged my sorry 30-year-old ass round the garden, picking up fag butts and half-empty beer bottles, surveying the ant colony setting up camp in the birthday cake remains, and realised I most definitely did NOT still have it. And I didn't bloody want it! What did the shorts get me other than an arse-full of mosquito bites? What good did a drink do? I didn't get drunk, I didn't have more than an hour's fun, and then I puked. Which I really hate to do. I could have puked in my baby's cot, for God's sake! It wasn't worth it. Not to mention the fact that everyone knew I'd gone to check on my baby and had then puked. This wasn't something I wanted circulating. It wasn't funny, I felt like my little bubble had been violated. I didn't fit there, *they* didn't fit here, and I didn't want to try and ram this square-peg me into the round hole of what life used to be like.

I couldn't do it anymore, I was too tired to fake it or try to do anything that required more prep than just turning up. It just wasn't working, this idea of what motherhood for a young woman was supposed to look like. I felt so miserable because I was caught between what I knew other people wanted for me, what I was in danger of missing out on and what I suspected was the only acceptable route for me at that moment: just sticking with my kid and not worrying about what was going on in the outside.

I was still scared to feed her in the evening, so I said good-night and lay in the bath with the monitor next to me, listening to her quietly grizzle in Rich's arms until she was asleep. Not one of the sleepless nights, the public shit explosions, the failed sexual acts or the bleeding nipples felt as bad as this. She didn't ask for me to be a total fuckwit! She demanded nothing, really. I had set up this routine for her and now was breaking it because I'd done something stupid, without thinking of the consequences. I blame the hangover for the histrionics, but also, mum guilt – a heady mix.

So, all in all, NOT a great birthday. But it was the first clue that maybe I was caught between the old me and the new me, and maybe I didn't much like my identity being in this state of purgatory. It might have been quite helpful since I didn't have friends to point it out, and everyone else – Rich, my parents – were too close to see it all unravelling so gradually.

I had spent decades building this person, readying her for work, love, friendships, but I'd been reformed in less than a year. I didn't recognise this woman, I wasn't sure Rich did either, and as for my friends – I had tried so hard to be unchanged but clearly, it wasn't to be. I flopped a wet flannel over my belly, sick of looking at it quivering in the water. *Rich is the same, why can't I be?* I thought of the way I saw my own mum – strident, powerful, a protector and friend – and wondered who my daughter would find in me. I felt pathetic, lost and utterly helpless.

I had turned 30. I hadn't worked properly this year other than writing some copy for a little-known skincare brand who were launching baby products, and probably thought I'd give them the *Vogue* spin on baby's arses.

My body, which I had rightly assumed would be in a constant state of flux, hadn't slimmed down as much as deflated and then sagged with the sheer exhaustion of it all. The cling-filmed ball of raw dough still hung forlornly between my hipbones. My boobs were still leaking but weren't big or round anymore. The stretch marks that had been so red and livid had faded to pearl-ised stripes of puckered flesh. This was it now – this is what I had to work with now.

My sex life was more of a sex death, and my social life was non-existent now Marianne and Lou were both back at work AND trying for more babies.

And our own baby was growing more and more independent. The breastfeeding that bound us in every sense was drawing to a close – I was already aware I was, for some people, heading into BITTY territory. I mean, nobody was more surprised than me that I was still breastfeeding.

I'd been fully immersed in the business of being a mum for a year, and loved it. But every time a milestone passed, the question pressed harder on me: as her reliance on me lessened, what else would I have to offer?

Coming up for air for a moment and stepping away from my mumness at my 30th had ended badly. Because I didn't want to be the person I used to be: I liked my responsibilities, I loved my baby. I didn't need to feel bad or unambitious for enjoying the quieter moments and the humdrum I'd been so frightened of. I was still me, there was still good in there.

CHAPTER NINE

RECOVERY

It all seems so obvious in retrospect, like it was the perfect time to dig deep and reinvent myself. The last few years had been a whirlwind of constant upheaval and with this new semblance of normality in place – sleep restored, more time on my hands, time to look in the mirror and think, WHAT THE FUCK HAPPENED?! Rich had decided to begin a Masters, he had started talking about moving house and what we might do next, a holiday perhaps. He was already planning adventures and questioning what would make us thrive while I was still stuck on the 'survive' setting.

If I'd been ready to accept that something was wrong, that something could be done to make life better for me and for the adults around me, who were either living on a knife edge depending on my mood (Mum) or doing a lot of Sudoku (Rich, Dad), I could have gently shaped a new me while I helped our toddler develop herself.

Instead, I basically went into hiding for a bit, convinced everyone had heard about puke-gate and thought I was a terrible mother and, more worryingly, a boring lightweight.

Because even a really posh gateau cake from Patisserie Valerie is no match for the mum puking on the rug. Everyone would judge this as the main talking point of any party. In reality, of course nobody cared, they didn't know I had secretly tried to rebrand as Earth Mother and they were used to puking at parties, I expect, but I was paranoid. I pretended my birthday had never happened, and resolved that since that part of me had to go, I'd just deny its existence and plough on as Earth Mother. I'd only do things that fit with this identity.

Oh, I'm a shouty mum

The problem was, Earth Mother wasn't cutting it now my child was becoming a toddler. She was a very reasonable toddler and we marvelled at how easy-going she was. But there were more challenging moments. Potty training. Tantrums. I felt like I wasn't heard a lot of the time, not by her or by Rich, and that I'd become the nag that drains the fun out of everything in the interest of getting to bed on time or eating up all the vegetables. Suddenly, I was swearing under my breath a lot, I was not as patient as I'd been for the months of mundane. I started to feel like a walking rulebook. It was so frustrating because I was aware what I was saying was boring and all the things I swore I'd never say – 'If you don't put that down right now, I'll …', 'I'm going to count to three and I want that coat ON, otherwise …'

I heard her reciting these same threats to her dolls one afternoon and realised the bits of my mothering she's soaking up are the bits that come so naturally to me but I'd sooner pretend never happened.

I thought I'd be so patient, I thought I could follow the books and do this thing with compassion, I'd think to myself, cursing myself for cursing. But actually I was still the woman who tsked dawdlers at Oxford Circus, who hated people who stood on the left-hand side, the impatient commuter. I was still me. DAMNIT!

I rushed through bath time and nagged her to get a move on when she was trying to engage me in one of her adorable games, which I then miss, and we inevitably argue. She was simply not as compliant – she's a person, after all – and I didn't seem to be as quick to anticipate her wishes and wants anymore. Just as the Earth Mother attachment parent bit had been a surprise, this polar opposite was equally shocking. I was wildly impatient and felt frustrated all the time.

I was desperate to do it *right*.

I was schooled by a fellow mum not to say 'no', but when I tried this I was so bogged down with trying to think of a way to rephrase 'NO, get down from that jagged rock or else you'll fall and crack your head open', that she fell off the rock and cracked her head open. Potty training at two was a nightmare as I got more and more impatient every time she wet herself, through no fault of her own. I hated the way I was doing it but it was SO hard to reign in the angry and be any other way. Who knew this stuff could be so frustrating? I nearly jacked it in several times, except that she could only start at our dream nursery in the spring if she was out of nappies.

Mum rages are unlike anything I've ever known because you don't WANT to feel it. If I'd been pushed to shout by anyone else I could have shaken it off, slagged them off to Rich until I felt justified in my behaviour. But when it's this child you love to distraction it hurts, because it feels like you're letting them down, and since they're the child you should always act like the best kind of adult, the adult they deserve. It was me I was pissed off with.

Raising a girl

I was also more aware that I was raising a girl suddenly. Until then she and her boy friends had been much of a muchness – they looked the same, their gender all padded out by nappies. But she'd deviated from the gender-neutral path we'd tried to set her firmly on and was asking me for a toy washing machine and ironing board, both in pink, please.

Raising girls seems to be far more different and specific to the gender than I'd expected, or at least it is for us. I can't help but pre-empt vulnerability to a greater extent than I do the boys around us. I am quick to make every learning curve into a diatribe on feminism and to empower her as a woman. I buy a lot of books that cast women in powerful roles, as well as the storybook versions of biographies of important women. She shrugs through most of them, not yet aware that women have to battle harder to have a voice, assuming still in her simple worldview that women and men are just the same thing, give or take a penis here and there. We bought gender-neutral toys, swore never to dress her in pink – and of course her natural instinct thus far has been to cradle her dolls and grab for the wands and princess dresses in the supermarket.

'What's your favourite colour?' I asked her one day, looking for reassurance that she has the beginnings of a feminist within her.

'Pink and blue.'

I inwardly high fived myself – see, gender neutral.

'I like pink Barbies and ponies, and blue tractors coz they're quite boy-ish,' she added. I began a 10-minute rant that picked apart this assertion, aware that I lost her about 15 seconds in, until she picked up her toy cars and shouted that we needed to put them in the bath immediately and I couldn't hear my own voice anymore.

I took her to so many coffee shops to avoid soft play that she orders her own babyccino now. She flashed her gummy grin and often stuck her tongue through her fingers in the international sign of licking pussies, because she did it once and of course we laughed. She told the postman, 'Mama loves Michael Bolton, you know?' even though I'd told her that was a secret.

She roared with laughter whenever my glasses slipped down my nose and when I drive she shouts 'Douchebag!' as the lights go red. Basically, she delighted in taking the piss out of me. And even though it's basically bullying, I loved it too.

I believed that I'd dress her like the kids in the White Company adverts, very 1940s evacuee meets short French eccentric.

ME: 'It'll be all Liberty prints and bloomers, won't it?'

REAL LIFE: 'Unlikely, babe.'

The reality now she can refuse clothes or rip them off is more Disney meets Sainsbury's TU in the 25 per cent sale, knock-off Crocs on her feet and a neon pink baseball cap on her head. I draw the line at Paw Patrol because they only have ONE female protagonist, but when she needs new pyjamas, who you gonna call?

That said, my tits don't jizz in the bath anymore. So, swings and roundabouts.

'Me time'

Aware that I could no longer hold my drink, I lived by the 'little and often' rule I think was supposed to apply to eating. Except that it was not that 'little' and it was VERY often. I got into a cycle of pouring a glass of wine as soon as the baby fell asleep, waking up feeling awful, drinking too much coffee and feeling poisoned, feeling even less patient, and come 7pm, cracking open another bottle.

Instagram was awash with crisply clean gin and tonics for what became the new cocktail hour (anytime after 4pm), the glass perspiring like a sexy Perspex phallus. Except that I no longer found phalluses sexy, try as I might.

I'm drinking too much, I thought, *and by not 'eating clean' I'm potentially robbing my daughter of having a healthy or even living mother past the age of 12*. Drink gave me the kind of buzz that almost felt like the old me, plus it's just for grown ups and I felt like I was being a naughty young woman again. *I deserve it!* I thought to myself, cracking open the third bottle of wine in a week. It was my independence, a mini escape and a nice treat. Until the second glass, which made me want to douse toast soldiers in leftover garlic and herb dip from Dominoes, before I passed out, dribbling and snoring into the sofa cushions in front of *Suits* or whichever other American series I was completely lost in. Ten minutes later, I would body-jolt awake, kicking Rich in the jaw, knocking the Dominoes sauce onto the rug. I would consider making a delicious, nutritious meal. I might eat a Ripple or consider a bath, but make do with a wee and collapse in bed, and troll people on Twitter who sleep well.

I also had to reconcile the fact that I was NOT a very good friend at that time – I've cancelled on nights out at the last minute because my baby didn't want me to leave or after an especially bad night's sleep; I couldn't hold a conversation or retain information in the way you'd like a supportive adult to do because my kid was also telling me something at the same time; I couldn't drop everything and just be there like I would have done before because it would have meant dropping a baby. Also, after a couple of years of trying to force it with women I had nothing in common with, and worse, women with kids who don't get on with my kid, I was less agreeable. Those are the worst – the play dates where you're constantly apologising because your kid hates every second of it but you know it'd be rude to cancel.

Maybe I'll just like, get a haircut?

I was brought up in the era of the makeover movie. As a kid in the 1980s you started with *Cinderella*, obviously – gets a new dress, moves up a social strata, escapes bonds of domestic slavery, finds love. Then when you're a bit older *Grease* tells you that a perm and a skin-tight black onesie will do the exact same thing if you're a dowdy frumpster with a bad fringe, 'lousy with virginity'. Even though I always thought Sandy was more beautiful before she transitioned to bad girl, this message was loud and clear: you didn't need to do that much work on your personality, it was all in the right accessories. *Moonstruck, Dirty Dancing, Pretty Woman* – all favourites, all undermining a woman's worth by requiring a better dress in order to succeed. The 1990s were wild for makeovers: *She's All That, Never Been*

Kissed, Clueless … And so as a teenager I wanted to pierce, tattoo and dye myself into an adult.

If you could endure the pain and the parental ear bashing to get your tongue/nose/lip/nip pierced, you were showing everyone how grown up but also edgy you were. I went for several in the ear – four of which were homemade, and three of which went through cartilage – and then my belly button when I turned 19. My mum was livid and didn't speak to me for a week, but I absolutely loved it. I also got blonder and blonder – I could be just the right shade of Britney without slimming down or getting new boobs, it was so easy!

I mean, I think I was justified in thinking a haircut and a tattoo might be the key to fixing some of the stuff that didn't feel right. To take back control without having to do very much or acknowledge what's behind these feelings.

If my ears were jangly enough, if my hair was pink enough and if I could just work out which tattoo I could cope with for the rest of my life, I could be a young woman again! I went back to the hairdresser I'd gone to pre-baby and told him I needed to dye the mumsy off me. My hair was sort of lank and floppy, constantly in a ponytail. I got blonder and then purple because I misunderstood my hairdresser's question, 'Lavender?' as pertaining to the scent of the shampoo, and murmured, 'Mmm, lovely,' and then had violet hair for two weeks. Ultimately, I settled on Millennial Pink because although I just missed that generation by a year, I figured I could fake it. That helped a bit, but it didn't last long and as we were living in a sleepy town in Sussex it didn't help me find my tribe because nobody else was doing it or remotely wanted to do it. Cutting it really short helped – *Look how brave I am! Cutting it all off so I have nothing to hide behind!* – because it showed off my neck, a body part unaffected by motherhood, and took less than three minutes to dry. Having an undercut made me feel like I was pretty badass. Years later, I read an obnoxious hairdresser in the *New York Times* coining the phrase 'mum hair' to describe a bob that shows little or no effort and certainly a total lack of style. Bastard.

The piercings couldn't stay because it hurt to sleep on them and I couldn't put up with anything extraneously interrupting sleep – the rewards simply weren't great enough. So I started thinking about tattoos. While I'd struggled in the past with finding the right design, suddenly there was this thing in my life that was everything I'd been looking for. *I could get her name,* I thought.

But someone beat me to it. No, not Rich: my mum.

One day she came in wearing the sort of smile she always wore when she'd done something ridiculous. She raised her wrist to my face and there, nestled by her watch, was my baby's name. Except without the accent. I. Was. Livid.

'It's so that it's the first thing I see when I wake up and she's always with me!' she crowed. This from the woman who had forbidden me from getting a tattoo because I'd go septic for sure and I would regret it but only for a minute because THEN I'D BE DEAD. And yet there she was, beating me to the post.

'You got … a TATTOO?!' I didn't even try to conceal how pissed off I was.

'Yes, but it's really sweet, isn't it? And it's sort of subtle, don't you think?'

'But … but … but, I wanted a tattoo and you didn't let me!!!'

'Hey, look, you can go to my tattooist –' *My mum has her own tattooist?* 'You can go and see Bill. I'll book you in and you can get one too.'

So now if I got a tattoo, it would be copying … my mum?! Here's me thinking it would be cool, a way to feel younger and tell everyone else I was younger, free, a bit rebellious. HOW IS IT REMOTELY REBELLIOUS IF YOUR MUM'S BEATEN YOU TO IT? It's not.

I still did it though, because by this point I'd pitched it as a story to *Red* magazine and I had a deadline. Two weeks to plan tattoo, get tattoo and write about tattoo, before having said tattoo photographed. My mum muscled in on this too, and so a photo shoot for two meant the piece went from being 'I am getting my first tattoo at 30!', a cool kind of zeitgeist thing where I could easily have been from East London and a member of Shoreditch House, to a pathetic 'My mum got a tattoo so I did too, even if it's smaller than hers, wahhhhhhh!'

I have a cute little 'Oof' on the underside of my right foot, 'Oof' being what I called the baby while she was in my tummy and also the only word I could get out during the worst moments of morning sickness.* But maybe I'm just not a tattoo kind of person. I am the person who will do anything for a byline though, it seems.

It was all part of me trying to reclaim 'mum face' as something cool and desirable, of trying to be young and fun. Actually,

---

* Annoyingly 'Oof' upside down in a French script looks remarkably like 'foot' without the 't'. As if I'd wanted to correctly label my body part but couldn't bear the pain to finish the word. Rich nearly died laughing when I got home and showed him.

my mum face was so many masks – a slick of unfeasibly bright pink lipstick to communicate I wasn't past it, bright blue eyeliner to show I was fearless and not struggling at all, a groomed brow to suggest I was groomed and not just made up of dry shampoo and Febreze.

The Mumpreneur

My brain was still set to Earth Mother, but one Saturday morning, Rich came back from the bank with some news.

'Our mortgage is up for renewal, bubs, and I've been saving up to pay a chunk off now.'

'WOAH! You've been saving up? And … wait, what?' I couldn't believe all this major stuff had just been happening and we hadn't discussed it. That I hadn't even thought to ask, or remembered where we were at with our mortgage. It later turned out I had been equally slack with my car insurance and MOT, but I pleaded the Fifth on that front.

'Bubs, you've been really busy with the baby. We haven't been spending as much so I thought it would be a good time to start saving for the future. It's not a big deal.'

'But I haven't … We always go halves on everything, I can't …' It was the first time we hadn't split everything big down the middle. I was broke because actually I *had* been spending a lot – coffee so the cafe owner didn't chuck me out mid-feed, new babygros when an al fresco shit is just too much for a single packet of Wet Wipes, a million breast pads, a gazillion nappies …

'Well, actually, you can do something. You've finally been self-employed for long enough to go on the mortgage now when we renew.'

When you go freelance you have no PAYE form that shows you're a good little earner. At the time we were applying for a mortgage to buy our cottage, you had to have three years worth of tax returns to show you did make money, and I was two years short, so Rich had to be the only name on the paperwork. Now I could finally step up.

'… Now she's nearly two, I thought *maybe* your mum could have her more often and you could … well, only if you want to. You need to have earned £7,000 by the end of your tax year in April.'

It didn't sound like much to have earned in a year but the sorry truth was I'd only managed about £2,000, monetising naps only when I wasn't comatose myself. I didn't feel stressed or upset though – I felt like he was offering me a role that was a bit more black-and-white than motherhood – it was just numbers and words which I had managed a thousand times before.

'I can do it, I can definitely do it. I'm going to do it, Rich.' The Earth Mother had to make it rain.

'You should start your own business,' Marianne said one day that autumn, as I panicked about earning £5,000 in six months. 'You should open up some kind of space that is about the mums, not the babies. No soft play, no shit tea, just comfy seats, proper coffee and loads of cake. You'd be good at making mums feel good.' I was really surprised she thought that. I confided I'd been thinking of creating something like that, but couldn't do it for real – I still struggled to do my buttons up in the right order.

'Don't be mad, of course you could do it. Think of all the things you've done! And I'd do it with you. We could do it together.'

So we did. I suddenly had all sorts of things to say that didn't start with, 'before I got pregnant'. It was making me feel quite powerful in a way.

'I'm really proud of you,' my mum tells me, squeezing my arm.

It was a success in that we had customers, got a bit of press and had our own blog (key to all mumpreneur businesses) but it did NOT make money. The first two months cost me £500. The next two barely broke even. The mortgage deadline was looming and I was using up the quota of babysitting time building a business that actually cost me money to run. I was not a mumpreneur after all; I had to rebrand quickly before I ran out of time.

Why does working feel selfish?

I threw myself back into pitching, and found I was actually a bit better at some bits of it than before. Having less time to devote to work meant I was picky, and only pitched things I desperately wanted to write. I was also way more focused – if I had a single nap time to write a whole feature, I'd damned well best get that feature written without a single side-step onto Twitter. I felt like a more efficient, less apologetic version of my old self.

I'm raising a girl, after all. I would approach work with the same attitude were she a boy, I know, but it seems doubly important that she sees me doing work I love, striving to improve and achieve. I want her to see me enjoying her and our time together *and* work. I wish everyday that I could still be happy not working and dedicating all of my time to her alone, but I've had to acknowledge however selfish it is, I can't. I do so much better when I have both. Of course, I'm lucky that my job works like that, that I can earn enough in that set up and that my mum is there to support that set-up – I'm painfully aware this career is hinged on so many predications swinging in my favour – but I mean to enjoy it while it's there, suck it and see.

I was also bolder. Back when she was about one and I was waiting for another Amazon Prime delivery of breast pads, tampons unravelling around my nipples in the meantime, I emailed Anna Wintour's Beauty Director at US *Vogue* to pitch a story. It had long sat on my wishlist of titles, but it took this change of perspective to make the first move. I think because if I did get knocked back, I expected to feel less of a knock – I had other stuff to take up the brain space that would formerly have swilled around the feelings of hopelessness and defeat at losing a big pitch or worse, embarrassing myself in the process. Fortune favours the brave though, and as it turned out, so does Anna. So I got to work on my first feature for *American Vogue*.

Victory, eh? I mean, I'm aware this sounds like it was all going pretty well. I was the brave favoured with the good fortune! BUT, in other respects motherhood had not, in fact, made me a better worker. For example, my brain was fried. It took so many attempts to write this admittedly very short feature on a new perfume, I was sweating bullets by the time I sent it in. I was also tired and lacked focus (see Chapter 7), and could only think of one word for perfume: perfume. I had the brief moments of nap time, a precarious set-up at the best of times, to knock out the piece that could make or break my career. Oh yeh, and my sense of perspective was back to being mental because we were midway through a nice bout of sleep regression.

Several transatlantic phone calls later I established the following:

'Anna doesn't like it.'

LIKE A STAB IN THE CROTCH AND BACK AND FACE!

Anna Wintour thinks you're shit! *But Anna, I did all this while nursing my baby until my nipples looked like earplugs! I have written it with a truncated labia! I am so tired!*

A call was scheduled, and of course the baby woke up just as the phone began to ring. I was forced to discuss WHY I couldn't articulate the intricacies of a mango and its creamy tang, with one nipple in a mouth and another being pulled by the pincer-like fingers of a tiny man-made sadist. I passed off the unavoidable yelps as my overwhelming enthusiasm for the opportunity. After a couple of these pseudo-torture phone calls, the piece was laid to rest and thank God came out in the magazine a few months later, edited to the point of being fairly unrecognisable. But my name was in *American Vogue*, so whatevs.

On the one hand, I was hustling when it suited me, and being at home with my daughter for the rest of time. On the other, work proved to be like a drug – the more I did, the more I wanted to do. I could feel the ambition pouring back into me. OK, so I had to work like I didn't have a kid and raise a kid like I didn't have a job. And reconcile the fact I'd be bad at both sometimes. A lot of the time, actually. And some days, I'd get really frustrated. If I make the fatal error of thinking I only need to be physically present and fire off emails from my phone, she gets cross and I achieve nothing. And of course even the best-laid plans fall apart on a regular basis.

It turned out I still LOVE working. I love feeling like a cog in a machine just as much as smashing through a to-do list myself. I love my job and writing was so much easier than talking in that first year because I could consider and edit myself as I went along. I could Google stuff and ask Rich, 'What's that word for when you need food and your belly gurgles?' 'HUNGRY?' 'Yes, actually I am, can you pass me a biscuit?' I could make sense of the world with words (when I could remember them), because they hadn't changed.

Having a baby had changed the way I wrote, though. Having a baby girl who would one day ask me what I did, made me ask myself, is it enough, just 'twittering on about lipstick' as one baby-group mum had summarised my career. I was already used to the difficult questions:

'Don't you feel bad plugging products that can't possibly work?'

'How do you feel about selling an impossible dream and making women feel bad about themselves?'

'How can you be a feminist and make out like make-up is important?'

Depending on who asked these questions, I wasn't that bothered because they clearly didn't know the kind of work I did. They'd probably never read my work. But I was less robust now. Would my kid be proud? This is what the knock to my sense of self and convictions had brought me to.

But do you know what? It is enough! I find myself on a mini crusade to use empowering language and turn the tide against self-esteem issues and racial discrimination and demonising the ageing process and instead towards self love. You know, one spot-busting how-to at a time. It's my little corner of the world that's all for me, and I'm good at it.

But wait – what kind of shit mum CHOOSES to spend time away from their kid?! I loved working so much and yet here I was, considering giving up precious hours with my baby to do something that 1. Didn't save lives, 2. Didn't benefit her in any obvious way. I'd always *had* to work – both because of the MORTGAGE and FOOD, and because I wanted to contribute – but here I was, upping the amount I would do, thinking about building my career back up, doing some kudos jobs and some strategic planning … I mean, sure, contributing to the household bills above the minimum meant we went from dire straits to slightly less dire straits (less eBay, more Ocado), but I still felt really guilty every time I had to palm her off on my mum, or when I willed her to go the fuck to sleep so I could finally get stuck into work. It turned out to be such a key part of bringing back some of my brain, my normality. Something familiar from before. I did it with a lot of huffing about having to bring in some money, etc., but ultimately, I loved every second of it, which of course made me feel awful.

So why does working feel selfish? Because of memes like, 'When in doubt, choose the kids. There will be plenty of time later to choose work'. Or even:

'You shouldn't value your work in the same way because that's selfish, that's not the way to nurture your children, who will inevitably be neglected. Even if you're putting in the minimum at work, it's really just time away from the kids'.

One of the things that has made me feel a bit 'fuck you!' about that is the very fact that NOBODY suggests Rich leaves his job to come home early. My work was always going to have to fit around childcare. Not because Rich is some kind of barbarian, but because his job was a constant source of income and mine was … sporadic. But I want my daughter to love her work, to find something that makes her happy like mine does, and to know that working is just as valid as leaving to raise kids. And to expect the same attitude from her partner. Also, um, I NEED THE MONEY! I need a house in which to have all the precious moments with said kid.

The kid started pointing at women in her picture books and telling me while rolling her eyes, 'She's going to work. AGAIN.'

And so I felt worse. But work gave me back an inner life where I wasn't ALL mum. I know lots of women who found this in running or going out again or travelling without the kids. For me, it was work. I told her all about it and one day she said, 'I'm going to write maza-geens and books like you. And I'm goinga be a BOOTY EDITOR.' And I felt a bit better.

Then just as my toddler turned two and we found a beautiful nursery that would welcome her as soon as she turned two and a half, I felt as though my workload might be ready for an upgrade. And by some miracle I was invited back to *Glamour* for a second stint as beauty editor, this time as the maternity cover for the girl who had replaced me. Oh, the circle of life, or rather, the workings of a female-dominated office. Just as the fog had begun to lift and I had begun to rebuild myself, the very same opportunity I'd had to forgo to become a mum had come up again. I had the opportunity to go back to where I was before this all began; after a very extended break I could just pick up where I left off and get back to it. I had another shot at the job I loved.

My first thought was 'No'. I can't leave the baby! I can't face the bright lights of the Big Smoke in my new wardrobe of smocked shirts and baggy leggings. I can't be a young person when I now look and feel 100. But I also really wanted to do it. The offer on the table was just one day a week in the office and another day from home. So that would be five days a week with the baby, a few hours at nursery and a few more with my mum. Could that be so bad? It was all starting to sound amazing, actually. And to have regular money coming in really clinched it. Finally the adventure was before me, one that I was familiar with and one that might bring me back to who I had been before. You know, without needing to puke on a rug. I was excited.

CHAPTER TEN

THE WORST NEWS

Things were definitely looking up. I'd accepted the job at *Glamour* in October, just as our baby turned two, but I wasn't due to start until February. Those two paychecks would take me up to my target for the mortgage man. We had Christmas ahead, the pressure was off, our girl was getting excited about nursery, and I started thinking about what our two lives would be like as we both tried new things. The endless cycle of care had started to ebb. She was entertaining everyone with her kind, wicked facial expressions and endless giggling. There was just more time at the end of each day to start considering, *what's next?* without feeling so guilty.

So of course another curveball was due, wasn't it? Because if there's one universal truth of parenting it's that just as you find your feet and feel confident enough to mix it up again, something will throw you right off course again, onto another mind-expanding trajectory. For most people, it's a second baby. You think to yourself, I've got this! I could do it again, because I know how it's done now and so we'd knock the sleeplessness and pain on the head this time. Look at this amazing child, we should do it all again! Let's have another baby!

Well, not for us. While everyone around us started to gestate afresh, we decided against it. No, it wasn't another baby that threw all the cards back up in the air: it was the threat of cancer.

One night when I was washing our two-year-old's hair, I noticed a lump on the back of her head. My fingers usually swept over the feathery hair of her scalp uninterrupted but this felt like a bump in the road. I immediately thought back to the moment a week before when she slipped on the bedroom floor. There were no tears, just a surprised expression that she quickly turned into a chuckle. *But had she banged her head? God, why do I have to be such a terrible mother?* I called for Rich to investigate. It was small – roughly the size of a Malteser, but soft and spongey to touch. He shrugged after she began to pull away from his hand, irritated.

'I don't think it's serious. If it was in her neck I'd say get it checked out, but it's probably nothing.'

'I'm going to take her to the doctor, anyway,' I say later that night when she's asleep and Google has thrown up nothing helpful about random lumps on the scalp of a two-year-old.

The GP gave the lump a token squeeze and said it was probably a glandular thing – perhaps she was fighting something off. Keep an eye on it, was the advice, and come back in a week if it's got bigger or if she had any other symptoms.

I buried the worry as soon as he gave a reason for it, except that a week later it was still there. Was it bigger, I wondered. I went back again, this time to a different GP at the practice, who agreed it was most likely a glandular thing that might take some time to disappear. With a packed schedule, however, the week flew by and the lump got bigger.

'I'm going back to the doctor's,' I told Rich. When he agreed, I knew I had cause for worry. He wasn't batting away my concern like he had when I thought a temperature might be the start of meningitis/sepsis/whooping cough.

The next GP said glands don't pop up on the head, so it might be a cyst, but not to worry, it would go of its own accord in time.

'If she gets a temperature or it starts to look red or feel hot, come here or to A&E to make sure it's not infected but it's so unlikely.'

Daft doctors who thought it was a gland, I thought to myself, *it's CLEARLY a cyst!*

We went up to see Rich's family and I wondered if they would notice the lump, now nearly golf-ball sized, peeking through the fine wisps of her hair. On our second night there, our kid was boiling hot. Sure enough, she had a temperature. The lump felt hot, as did the rest of her tiny body. We organised to see the out-of-hours GP in the hospital up the road that night. I could feel everyone shaking their heads behind me – here she goes again, that nutbag, overreacting, overthinking everything.

'No, it's not infected – this is a really benign cyst, I've removed hundreds,' the young doctor in A&E drawled, rolling his eyes at me. 'The temperature is nothing to worry about – probably just a virus. See your own GP when you get home and they'll most likely get it removed.' It was clear he felt we were wasting his time.

We returned home the next day and I made another call to the GP – the skin over the bump looked strained, it had grown harder.

'It's not infected, but I'm going to refer you to a paediatrician,' the GP said, after she'd called a colleague in to have a feel of the lump as well. 'Now, I don't want you to worry – I'm not worried,' she said, giving me the Kind Eyes look, 'but let's just make sure we've ticked all possible boxes so you can relax. You should get an appointment in the next couple of weeks.'

I decided to call Pete, a dermatologist friend. If it was a cyst, perhaps he could put our minds at rest sooner in the comfort of his cosy consulting room. We took her there confident that he'd send us on our way feeling free of the worry, as he'd done with several of my dodgy moles over the past few years. We didn't imagine for a second he'd be more worried than us.

'This isn't a cyst,' he said straight away, moving a light over her head as she patiently sat under his probing fingers, looking to us for reassurance. 'I want you to go and see my friend John, he's an excellent radiologist and can look at what's inside the lump.'

I still didn't think the worst. Even when he rang us back with an appointment for the following day, not trying to cover the sense of urgency in his voice, I didn't clock it. I imagined they'd drain it and worried what this would mean for the hair over that spot. Can you even put a sticking plaster on their heads, or would it rip the hair out? Oh God, would they have to shave it? She would hate that …

Rich came down from his office in the physiotherapy department to meet us outside radiology and everyone was quite jolly. The radiologist passed an ultrasound over her head – it was just like the one used to find her in the depths of my belly, and now we were routing around in her skull to see what else we could find. A student doctor hovered by the screen as John pointed out the various dimensions of the lump with words I couldn't understand.

'Might be a haematoma – has she had a fall or bumped her head recently?'

'No, and it's been growing steadily for the past six weeks,' I answered quickly.

'I think we need an X-ray,' he finally said.

I looked at Rich – aren't X-rays for bones? Why are we looking at the bone? And I went back to the moment in the bedroom when she'd slipped. Had her skull fractured?

We were ushered into another waiting room and moments later, an X-ray technician came out to us, and told us that just one of us could accompany her.

'I'll go,' said Rich, 'I think it'll stress you out.' I squeezed her chubby little leg, kissed her hand, and with that they were gone. Standing alone in this small anteroom it suddenly hit me that this could be a moment. I felt sick, I started to shake. I was breathless. I wanted to break into the X-ray room. I wanted to pull her off the table and go home, put that old familiar nursery rhyme CD on, pull down the blinds, blank it all out. It felt so wrong to be out here when she was in there, going through something. But Rich was right – he was calm and steady and she would find more comfort in that. In my head I began to recite, 'Lavender's blue dilly dilly, lavender's blue, if you love me dilly dilly, I will love you …'

They were in there for ages. I texted a friend, my fingers twitching, 'They've taken her in for X-rays, I don't know what's going on, but I think it's bad.'

When they finally came out, John was telling Rich not to worry. Rich smiled wanly at him and my stomach dropped.

'I think he's saying it's cancer,' he whispered as we walked quickly along the corridors. It was by far the worst thing I have ever heard anyone say in my entire life. My hairline prickled and my limbs felt both heavy and empty. I was careering down the corridors as if we could run away from it. Inside I was screaming, *What-the-fuck, what-the-fuck, why-why-why-why?* I needed to know everything and I needed the reassurance Rich had always been quick to give, but nothing was coming out of his mouth as he tried to process everything and keep our daughter blessedly unaware. We talked with fake smiles plastered on our faces so she wouldn't sense any ill. Which is weird, of course – imagine discussing your daughter's possible cancer, the worst fucking thing that has ever happened to you, with a clownish grin on your lips and your voice light and breezy. It went a little something like this:

'What the fuck do you mean, they *think* it's cancer, what is it? Is it cancer or not?' I asked in a singsong voice, that smile wobbling slightly on one side.

'He doesn't know yet but he thinks it might be like some form of cancer, hahahaa!' Rich gave a wide-eyed chuckle, as the kid looked up at him curiously.

'What now then, babycakes?' I asked him – I had never called him that before, but the false levity was confusing me.

Eventually we reached the car again.

'I'll be home in just a couple of hours, bubs – will you be OK?' I nodded, unable to look at him, smiling instead at her, sure I was about to die right there in the car park. I cried all the way home, silently so she wouldn't know, the nursery rhymes louder than ever on the car stereo.

That night my friend Pete, the dermatologist, rang us. It wasn't good. He kept telling us over and over how sorry he was, that he didn't know much about the disease John had semi-diagnosed, but he'd read up and thought radiotherapy might help. Might help?! No 'don't worry' platitudes, just pity and radiotherapy. It felt hopeless.

I drank a very strong pint of gin and tonic and cried for hours on end, Rich occasionally joining in. I couldn't breathe, I couldn't sit still or be comfortable.

Her toys lay on the rug in front of us, and I felt like she was already dead as they went untouched. I saw the hole she would leave, every item in the room touched by her or bought for her. I imagined everyone I knew crying. What would the other mums say, as they clutched their own children to their chests and sobbed over the injustice, thinking themselves so lucky? I wondered what my mum would do, imagining it would kill her outright if I told her. She'd want to surround us with crystals and take us to homeopaths and the very thought made me angry. I couldn't stop thinking of my baby's tiny fingers falling limp, her perfect skin as yet unmarked by the wicked world, and her kind, curious eyes closing. Rich began researching the name we'd been given – this disease that affects just one child – *our* child – in hundreds of thousands of kids.

I literally couldn't give two shits about anything else anymore. The issues I'd been going through with friends, sex, work, the size of our house, the size of my belly, how much money we didn't have, what people thought of me – it was all forgotten as I was thrown into this new reality where we were just trying to keep our heads above water, paddling frantically and looking around for help. I didn't care who I was or how I'd changed, all I could feel was panic and a desperate need to keep my child safe. It was a primal feeling – I was suddenly all nerve-endings and fight, nothing more. I'd have *killed* for a worry over shoes or haircuts. This was so fierce it had overridden every other instinct and thought.

We agreed that night that I wasn't resilient or sensible enough to be allowed to research it myself. Google had already suggested I was dead countless times in my own research as a bona-fide hypochondriac and Rich said there were articles just waiting for me that would surely drive me further into the depths of despair. 'You go straight to the worst-case scenario with that stuff, so isn't it best to find out what's happening to her from an expert, not what *has* happened with other people?' he suggested. 'I could give you stats and survival rates but we have no idea which end of the spectrum she's on and so they won't help us know what she has ahead of her, I promise.'

I knew he was right – Google was not my friend. So I used Rich as a conduit. He fielded the salient information my way, and I knew nothing more. I know how it sounds, but it worked for us.

Instead of doing mind maths with the stats and seeing phantom symptoms in her, I waited for our appointment with the paediatrician, who John had already contacted to update them with a diagnosis. OK, so I did work out what the consultant's email address would be and sent her lists of my concerns and worries (I had to try various formats – have you ever tried finding a doctor's email address online?! It's nigh on impossible! And now I know why …). But otherwise I left well alone and tried to stop thinking about what kind of funeral we'd have for our daughter. I did Google the doctor though, and saw she specialised in childhood oncology. Cancer then, even though John and Pete had been a bit vague as to whether this illness constituted cancer or not; it seemed we had our answer.

We decided it would be better to keep the news to ourselves rather than tell either set of grandparents. If Rich thought letting me loose on Google would be a bad idea, the thought of fielding their questions and reactions and fears was overwhelming. And to be honest, I couldn't tell anyone because it would ground it in reality and indelibly mark it as a moment in our families' history. It would become part of our daughter's story whereas if we kept it under wraps, life could continue either side of it, and nobody would look at her with pity or let on to her that they were sad or scared. It would be easier to keep up this façade for her that all was fine. Life could go on, with only the evenings Rich and I found ourselves alone to fall apart.

'I love you, baby,' I told her, roughly a million times in one day.

'I love cheeeeeeeeeeeeeese' was generally her reply.

I wanted to take that fucking lump and stick it in my own head, to fight it with my body and show it the full force of my rage. I wanted her to have a regular sick bug and vomit all over me, so I could clean it all up and pop her in clean crisp sheets with freshly washed hair, make her feel better. What hurt is that the cure wasn't in finding her a great nursery, buying her new toys, taking her for a wholesome walk on the beach, feeding her Calpol, or even breastfeeding – nothing I had in my arsenal was going to be good enough. In fact, why the fuck had I breastfed so long for? Why had I obsessed over this healthy, organic and sugar-free diet for her? Where had it got her? All those people who had told me it was so worthwhile and her immunity would be so strong! I wanted to call them and tell them it was *too* strong now, so thanks for nothing. I wondered if the anti-nausea medication I'd taken during my pregnancy had caused this, or if my mum had been right all along and mobile phones really do cause cancer. I should never have used my phone while I was feeding her – by hovering it above her head as she suckled I had probably zapped her brain and caused this whole trauma myself. I couldn't sleep or eat, or talk to anyone.

On Saturday, Rich insisted we still take her to her baby swim class. We were surrounded by people who didn't know and it actually felt good to escape into an alternative reality where everything was fine, normal, just as it had been the previous week. As we were about to leave, she staggered backwards from the sliding doors, as if she'd bumped her head. I caught her up in my arms and saw her eyes were rolling back in her head. I screamed at Rich, 'She's having a seizure, she's having a seizure!' The couple alongside us continued to put their toddler's shoes on, respectfully averting their eyes as this unfolded, but I didn't care who heard it. Rich snatched her away and checked her over, and then hurried outside to the car, me running after him, carrying our shoes. We drove straight to A&E, even though as I looked at her in her car seat she was fine again.

The nurse had never heard of her illness, but said he'd start by checking her over before investigating. He explained it seemed like she had poked herself in the eye and was rolling her eyes because it was the instinctive way to try and lubricate when you've poked yourself.

'So we brought her to A&E because … she poked herself in the eye?'

I couldn't look at Rich as I said this, but the nurse smiled.

'Look, you're on high alert, and you're welcome to come back anytime you think something is wrong. Anytime. Honestly, it's fine.'

We left feeling relieved but I couldn't shake the feeling that this kind of drama wouldn't have happened before this all began. What this illness had already done was to take away Rich's voice of reason. I'd been talked down from worst-case scenarios by Rich so many times, I had grown to believe it was genuinely unlikely anything bad would ever happen to our daughter. But he had been wrong. How could I ever trust him again? We had gone to A&E because of a poked eye, we had both jumped to the worst-case scenario. Suddenly, the dynamic of neurotic wife and laid-back husband had been smashed and I felt vulnerable to a hundred worst-case scenarios with no way of climbing down from this window ledge. A sword was literally dangling over our heads, and I suspected it would be there for the rest of our lives.

I realised that the first appointment with the cancer specialist would be pivotal. Depending on the way she spoke to us – solemn and hushed tones vs. positive, upbeat and dismissive – I would find my new mindset. I'd be analysing every word and sigh with the vehemence of a high-school crush.

First off, the doctor was abrasive. But I took this as a good sign – you're never going to be mean to someone you're about to tell is going to lose their child, right?

She checked our kid's body from head to toe, massaging every inch of her with her eyes focusing upwards as she scanned for more lumps. I didn't want to distract her – I wanted her to be thorough – but I had to ask:

'Is it cancer?'

'Not cancer, no. It sort of depends how you define "cancer" – yes, it's cells going rogue as they do in cancer. Plus, it's sometimes treated with chemo, which is why oncologists treat it. But no, this isn't cancer.'

It was not cancer. And by the way, I'm not going to share the name of the illness with you now, for three reasons. The first is that I know what I need to know; I still haven't Googled it once, and I can't have you knowing more than me. I have to trust that only the doctors know more than we do, and that's a safe scenario for me, because I know even the best people – the best friends – can say the wrong thing and I'd be undone. The second is that we don't know for sure what it was, of course. Finally, it's my daughter's story, should she ever wish to tell it. Just as I can't have you knowing more than me, nobody should already know more than her. It might seem selfish, but I don't want it to be inextricably linked with her name, nor do I want any of us to be faced with cases worse than hers, with examples of what could have happened. I never want to have to think of it again.

Anyway, NOT cancer. But in case you thought I'd be whooping for joy, she'd just floored me with another C-word I dread: chemo. You're going to chemo my kid? So, it's just cancer with an alias, then – it's like when Prince tried to change his name to a symbol but people were still like, 'Who? Oh, you mean Prince!'

She said at the moment the chances of needing chemo were seriously unlikely. We didn't know it was that for sure, and anyway, it was just one small lump. She was definitely talking the whole illness down. She was using a level tone, dismissing the kookier of my questions – will her skull collapse and crush her brain, will she lose motor skills, would she still be allowed to drive and operate heavy machinery?

The doctor had seen one similar case the previous year and once they'd treated it, it hadn't returned. That child had recovered and was free, so it was possible we would be too. And it turned out that the treatment wasn't as bad as we'd feared either. Usually by taking a scraping of the bone wherever the lump had appeared, you triggered a healing process that would knit the bone back together and heal the hole caused by the rogue cells. No radiotherapy, and no chemo.

I felt like I'd won something, like we'd been dipped into the fiery depths of hell but were now jumping on a Virgin flight to – maybe not heaven, but … Magaluf? I wouldn't have chosen to go there, but wouldn't sniff at it now. Not Heaven because there was still the small matter of a head-to-toe X-ray, blood tests and urine samples to check her organs were unaffected and there were no other lesions. So, still a big whack of uncertainty. Then there was the biopsy. She referred us to an oncologist in Southampton, because dealing with my baby's perfect baby-sized head counted as neuro-surgery, which took place at a bigger hospital.

In the meantime, we went home happy that it was almost-not cancer. The operation wasn't so invasive – nothing was being removed as such and that would most likely be the end of it all. Suddenly having a tiny piece of her removed didn't seem like such a drama compared with what we had faced before – it's weird how quickly your brain adapts and changes the trauma-score of previously inconceivable torture. It's a moveable scale.

Leading up to the next appointment, we noticed the lump was suddenly disappearing. It was no longer protruding, and the day we visited Father Christmas in his grotto, I realised I couldn't feel it at all. Had I mentioned it was Christmas? Oh yes, the most wonderful time of year. We were holding this dark secret in while singing carols and forcing mince pies down our necks. Tra la la la la, la la la la.

On 20 December we went to Southampton. I don't know what I'd expected but when we were buzzed into what turned out to be a children's cancer ward, I felt my throat tightening. There was a list of first names on a white board opposite the small bank of seats, some of which had clearly been scrawled by children. Ethan, Kaylie, Sam … they all had cancer.

We were directed to a cheerful but awful playroom, a bit like the nurseries I'd looked round, full of toys, books and a TV playing *CBeebies*. A door to the left was marked 'School Room', and kids' drawings were given pride of place all over the walls.

'It's really clean, I guess to protect the kids whose immunity is low,' whispered Rich. 'It's like your ideal playgroup.' I know it was an attempt to make light of the situation but even the thought of a sanitised playroom couldn't cheer me up. A tall toddler in just a nappy dashed from toy to toy and eventually sat down to do some colouring alongside us. I joined his mum on the sofa as Rich passed out crayons.

'So, what kind of cancer has she got?' she asked gently. I said I didn't know yet, that we were just at the beginning, because I couldn't bear to tell her it was nothing more than a tiny hole in her skull and the biopsy alone was probably as far as we'd go. This woman and her son were 18 months into three years of treatment for leukaemia. He'd never grown hair as he'd gone in as a baby and would leave as a child ready to start school. But she was convinced he would leave. She didn't seem depressed even, just another tired mum who bemoaned his manners and told brilliant stories about the cheeky words he used and how funny he could be at bath time. I asked where they lived.

'Right here. We have to be here all the time, so my husband lives back at our house with our other son, and I live here.'

Finally, it was our turn and the mum smiled in the way that every mum at every baby group had smiled at me, bridging the gap between strangers who would hopefully become friends, bonding over our kids.

Our new doctor gently examined our now slightly fractious kid.

'Mama, she has babies in her belly.' The doctor – who definitely did NOT have a baby in her belly – chuckled and carried on. I tried to laugh with her but it came out as a growl-vomiting sound.

'I can't see any signs of other lesions and the fact that this one is receding is such a good sign,' she said. She was the first person we'd seen who was fully confident in how the disease worked and she was full of good news. The first was that it was absolutely not a cancer, and it was only treated with chemo in rare cases. And it seemed unlikely she'd need that, given the lump was going away of its own accord. Most were self-correcting, and had we not been referred, we'd probably never have found out. Life would have continued without interruption. I chose not to focus on that fact for long, except to soak up the positive side like a sponge.

Suddenly the dark future we'd seen looming before us was no longer a fait accompli. We were unbelievably lucky and that was an amazing feeling after weeks of terror. And it came so easily. It took one woman to put us on another path, to remove the danger. We still had the full body X-ray – booked for 29 December – and then the biopsy, but we were one step closer to feeling far better. Plus, we were going home for Christmas.

I felt guilty leaving, though. I know the parents looking at us thought we'd be taking up the neighbouring bed. And then we left. My face crumpled up as we walked through the heavy doors into the austere corridor, a Tupperware tumbled from my bag as we swept through.

'Leave it,' Rich gruffly whispered, pushing me forward, not letting me show my pity to the parents on the other side. It didn't feel like a place wrought with death, but the suffering was visceral.

So we hit the M1 with all the presents, treats and sense of impending doom with which most families approach Christmas. When we stopped for petrol midway, I picked up a voicemail from the hospital – the biopsy was scheduled for 2 January.

Christmas was fucking awful. I couldn't relax and every time she looked hot or made a face I had to check her all over. I kept looking at her fine hair, her smooth skull and imagining it all being chipped away. I knew everyone thought I was acting crazy but I didn't even try to suppress it anymore. It got really dark inside my brain – would this be our last Christmas together? Would she start nursery in the spring? Would she get to grow up? Then she stopped peeing and I remembered that the doctor had warned diabetes could take hold when the organs are affected.

On Boxing Day she had a temperature and still wouldn't pee. We went to A&E, where the doctor drew a blank when we mentioned her illness's name – Rich told him not to Google it, obviously – but duly tested her urine and said nothing was wrong. Keep her cool, was his advice, and as we left the strip-lit hallway, we saw it had snowed. I drove around the cul-de-sac until she fell asleep and then sat with her while she napped in my mother-in-law's bed, stroking her forehead. I knew it wasn't doing much for my reputation as a crazily neurotic mum, but I just wanted to be with her in peace. Being alone with her made it all stop for a moment: I could see she was alive, I could focus on her chest rising and falling.

We went home and 29 December arrived at last. We were back in hospital for the tests, trying to convince her the sticky numbing gel they put on kids' hands pre-needle wasn't evil. She cried inconsolably. I thought about all the needles and X-rays she'd endured, and somehow this gel was the thing she hated most.

'Could we just do it without the gel?' I asked a nurse.

'It'd be really traumatic for her, love. And a nightmare for us to get the needle in.'

I looked at our daughter's little face, lower lip wobbling as she waved her hands around, trying to shake off the stickers they'd placed over the gel to stop her wiping it off.

The play therapist tried to distract her with a Peppa Pig game, but she was too smart for them – craning her neck to see what was happening with the arm they'd pulled behind her for the phlebotomist. He was being coaxed to the chair by a nurse who was clearly trying to help him steady his nervous hands. In the end I barked at him to get on with it so we could leave, and they drew the blood as she sobbed into my neck.

The urine test was another version of hell, too. We'd only just finished potty training a month before so she was routinely withholding pee until it just seeped out of her unannounced. I sat her on the toilet five times, cup poised beneath her, elbow-deep in the bowl of a hospital toilet. They have one loo in the children's assessment unit. ONE!

Then came a whole hour spent trying to get X-rays of each part of her body, from her wriggling shoulders to her tiny toes. This time we both insisted on being there and I acted like a maniac, trying to entertain her while Rich pinned her to the table. We were warned about exposing ourselves to radiation, but with our tiny kid lying there with it poised over every part of her, it seemed like the most ridiculous warning. I was torn between not wanting to traumatise her and wanting to get it over with as quickly as possible so we could get back to being average Joes, watching shit kids' TV and feeling guilty about the fish-finger lunch.

Instead, we sat in the waiting room, not sure what we were waiting for. John soon appeared and was so obviously happy we didn't even make it to his office before he said, 'There's nothing else there! AND the original lesion in her skull we found three weeks ago has nearly totally disappeared!' I felt my knees buckle and I cried hot, happy tears. We went home and put on carols and ate mince pies, my little girl blissfully unaware of what we were celebrating but enjoying the belated Christmas.

Our oncologist called the next morning to cancel the biopsy – it was decided no further treatment was necessary. We'd go back to Southampton for a check-up in the spring, and then she said it would be a yearly appointment.

It was over. The whirlwind stilled inside me.

We still don't know for sure what it was, but are content that it's caused no problems and if it was what they would have been testing for with a biopsy, nobody thought it necessary to know. It wasn't such a threat that we couldn't just let her body do its thing. I was in awe of the strength and clout of this tiny body that had knitted itself back together without any assistance. She's a superhero, she fought off a beast, probably while sat slack-jawed, watching Mr Tumble arse around. I hope she'll be as proud of her body as I am.

CHAPTER ELEVEN

RELAPSE

We survived the biggest earthquake, and at first I was high as a kite. But then I realised it was taking longer to shake off the aftershocks. No matter how many times I relived the moment we knew she was going to be absolutely fine, I also had the scariest moments of my life playing through my mind's eye like a vignette. I repeat SHE IS OK over and over like a mantra and it cools the boiling to a gentle simmer.

Things get really shit

I wish I could look back on the darkest days and say things like, 'It put things in perspective,' and 'It made me not sweat the small stuff.' But it absolutely didn't. OK, *some* of the bigger things that would have floored me before fell away a bit – I had no regrets when friendships failed because I was mainly concerned with my unit of three. I didn't worry about what people thought of me so much. I wasn't so acutely aware of the things we didn't have and couldn't afford. But the small stuff? I still sweated it plenty. In fact, while we're on the subject, do you know what *really* pisses me off? The way a Bag For Life nearly ALWAYS loses its handle in the first year of use. Their lifespan is briefer than a hamster's, for fuck's sake.

I appreciated how miraculous my kid was, just like the newborn days. She was kind, she was funny and she was really getting into her stride with swearing, so it was just getting better and better. We were out having lunch with another family of three, and the kid was being kind of shy. She eked out her friendliness in small, random portions and usually only when she was impressed by someone. The dad was telling her knock-knock jokes and she was not laughing. *It'll take more than that, sunshine,* I could almost see her thinking. Finally, he gave up.

'OK, well, what's the funniest thing you've ever heard?'

She pondered this for a moment, the whole table goes quiet and braces itself for a cute moment, perhaps a little 'Doctor, Doctor!' joke or her favourite skit from *Hey Duggee*. She looked up at the ceiling, deep in thought, until finally:

'Probably ... shit-bags?'

Interestingly, the frustrations didn't just disappear. I didn't find myself suddenly thinking, *you know what – she can do what she likes, I am just glad she's alive*. OK, I did for a while, but then real life started back up again. It didn't make me more patient, which I could have sworn it would when we were in the ugly depths of it all. I still cared about fulfilling my ambitions, I still bickered with Rich about who should go up when she wakes in the night, I still got cross when she dawdled at bedtime or wouldn't eat her supper. It's crazy how quickly your brain slides this uncomfortable yet life-affirming truth to the sidelines, and you start to worry about the meaningless shit again. And thank God we have the luxury of worrying about such things. Because

I'd take angst over who's due a lie-in and which day the bins are collected over illness any day.

I thought I was less fun with her than Rich. It fell to me to keep things going, to coax her to eat, dress, sleep, bark out orders, chivvy her through our routine. I was aware Rich was the fun one – he came home from work and they played, with me occasionally begging him to keep things calm and … well, boring in the lead-up to bedtime. I heard them thundering across the hallway upstairs.

'Come on, Dada! Let's be lions eating a steak!'

'YES! OK, what kind of steak? Reindeer? Beef steak?'

'NO! FUCK'S STEAK!'

Rich came down smirking and told me I might want to dial down the swearing around her, for the eleventy-billionth time.

I thought that if I told myself 'If your kid is healthy, nothing else matters' so often, I'd begin to feel it. One friend I said this to mistook what I meant by that:

'So it's chocolate finger sandwiches for supper then?' she joked gently, knowing I hadn't allowed anything containing refined sugar in the house since day dot.

But that's not what I meant. That stuff still matters if it's what you believe will benefit your kid. What I ACTUALLY meant was that I no longer cared how anyone *else* feels about what I'm doing here as a mum. Sure, I still experience self-doubt about the way I do things on a daily basis. But I have let go of the buzz of feedback. Think I'm a bore because she's not yet allowed sweets? Fine. You offended that I cancelled our play date because she seems tired? Your problem. I will never again go through with a play date just because I don't know how to say no. I will never again put up with an obnoxious child whose own parent won't step in. I will put my kid before everyone else, before what other people think of us. I will put my kid before my social need to people please. I will not sweat the friends I've lost because they didn't get it.

I also learned that while the process of having a baby and that newborn stage can create camaraderie with other men and women, as if bound together in wartime laughing about the darker sides of parenting, a disaster like this is totally isolating. Nobody will say the right thing; nobody will understand your angst and pain. I learned that the worst can indeed happen, despite your best efforts to rage against it.

She didn't have cancer. She didn't have an ounce of treatment. If I hadn't persevered we might never have known she had anything out of the ordinary. LET'S NOT BLOODY CONSIDER THAT FOR LONGER THAN A SECOND THOUGH, GUYS. But still – the threat of real-life trauma was revealed as something we couldn't escape. It wasn't something we'd watched from afar and shook our heads in solemn disbelief when it happened to other people – it was something that could happen to any of us at any time. I didn't trust the good news as resolutely as I had the bad – Rich and the majority of GPs were like the bucket of sand you keep near an open fire – I could dollop a good chunk of their superior knowledge and rational thinking on my neurotic worries. Now? Not so much. My neurotic worries had been accurate so now how could I possibly trust Rich when he tried to convince me a temperature and a common cold wasn't actually meningitis? How could any GP discount Lyme disease before we'd seen a consultant?

From then on, every lump, bump and raised gland in our kid was terrifying. And over the next two years I'd undergo a mammogram, colonoscopy, four smear tests, countless blood tests and more than one mole check. We can never watch *Thomas The Tank Engine* again because that was the kid's show of choice through that terrible month and now the theme tune triggers panic attacks in me, and the Southampton Ikea is dead to me because the whole city now gives me the willies.

'Rich, I've had wind for, like, two days now. I think there's something really wrong.'

'Right. So you think that fart might be cancerous?'

'Yes, I do actually. Because also, last week I also had quite an urgent poo, you know?'

'Yes, I remember you telling me. I wish I didn't. So you'll go to the doctor again and tell them what? That you farted? Because admittedly, Grace, it was bad but I don't think bad enough for another colonoscopy.'

'But what about the bowel movement, too? I mean, the symptoms are totting up.'

'But of course someone actually already checked didn't they? Someone literally put a camera up your arse to check it was OK up there. And did they find cancer?'

'Well, no, but –'

'That's great then! No cancer! Your arse is fine.'

Every day when Rich came home I would try to mime symptoms and rashes out to him over the kid's head so she wouldn't know I was worried. He was patient at first, but became increasingly fed up.

'The worst thing would be if this episode – which, by the way she is totally unaware of – ended with you making her paranoid about her health, Grace. If she ended up as nuts as –'

'AS NUTS AS????'

He didn't finish this sentence because he is never one for a row. But I was seething and also worried he was right.

Rich kept telling me to lock it down – don't show her any fear, don't obsess over her health, stop being so scared – but as I tried to push it down it felt like I would explode, like nobody could hear me even though inside I was screaming bloody murder.

Things get even shittier

I decided I wouldn't go back to *Glamour* after all. *How can I? I am the vigilant one; I know what to look for. If six GPs missed the true cause of this bump, how could anyone else be trusted with her care?*

I also decided she shouldn't start nursery either. I mean, all those kids, all the pushing and shoving. The teachers only needed to take their eyes off her for a minute and her fragile little skull could be crushed, or she might lose an eye.

Also, I stopped drinking coffee and tea because they made me more anxious. I started crying as soon as she'd gone to bed and rarely let up much before 11. Rich started going to bed early, his face blue in the light of his laptop. We didn't speak.

One morning the bill for the first term of nursery arrives.

'Bloody hell, there's a deposit in here too – what, do they pay that back in a couple of years if she hasn't broken anything?' Rich was digging around in The Messy Drawer for his chequebook.

'Don't need to pay that,' I mumbled, 'she's not going.'

'Bubs,' Rich sighed but didn't look up, 'Not this again. She needs it – she's old for her year and she needs to hang out with other kids, we agreed. If she'd been born just a few weeks earlier she'd be starting school soon. And you start your new job soon – your mum can't be expected to do all the childcare on her own.'

'I'm not going to do the job anymore. I've told them she's ill.'

Rich looked up, a pained, strained and exhausted look on his face.

'She's not ill, though, is she?' He was quiet. The kid was in the living room next door watching TV, mesmerised by the *Twirlywoos*.

'I can't let her go, Rich, she's not ready. What if –'

'GRACE, IT'S ALREADY HAPPENED! The worst has already happened! And you were there, you were there every day. Nothing could have stopped it – not you, not your breast-feeding or your worrying. You can't control it all now, and we probably never did!'

'She's not ready, if you could just –'

'YOU are the only one who isn't ready. This isn't fair on her, it's not in her interests. Look, she's my kid, too, and it feels like you're doing what you think will make YOU feel better. The fact is YOU will damage her if you don't move on and bloody LET IT GO. Let her be a normal kid. She IS going to nursery.'

A key rifled in the lock and my mum blew in with the wind, laden with bags.

'HELLOOOOO! Where's my baby?! GG's here so Mummy can go have some nice reflexology, let's PLAY!'

Damnit, she's caught her watching TV again, I realised, as Rich stalked off to the bathroom to get ready for work.

CHAPTER TWELVE

A NICE FOOT RUB

Pat was holding my right food firmly between her warm hands. Apparently the left foot was a no-go since verrucae ARE kind of a deal-breaker for a reflexologist after all, so I just asked her not to make me emotionally lopsided with her rubbing.

I had been feeling lost for years now but the feeling was broken up into fractured pieces – friendships, my body, my career, my marriage – and it was only when Pat, the reflexologist, pieced them together for me that I saw it was me that was broken. Rich hadn't changed a whole lot, my friends hadn't changed, our families were rolling with the punches I'd been lobbing at them on and off for the past three years. When I added up all the parts of me that were lost in the processes of bringing up a baby, it all made sense.

My sense of self was still in a constant state of flux. Every time I thought I had a grasp on motherhood, the rug was pulled from beneath me – teething, weaning, nursery, sleep training, growing pains, illness, tantrums, separation anxiety, potty training, first swear words … Nothing is constant.

Then just as things started to fall into place – like Dorothy's house coming down from the twister in Kansas – that terrible diagnosis forced my identity crisis into sharp focus. And everything sped up again. But I was still here, lagging behind, hollering for everyone to slow down and let me catch up.

Before I got pregnant, being in control was my thing and my day was timetabled – like most working women's – so that there was a clear boundary between work and relaxation. Now it's all work and the only play is the kind that involves Barbies and Duplo bricks. And society's telling me, now I'm a mum, that's all I am.

I don't want to accept this, to feel like I'm done, like I'm over. That my narrative is at an end as hers begins. I don't want my daughter to discover photos of me as a young woman and not recognise me, find it unimaginable that I had adventures once upon a time, stories and a life she struggles to equate with the me she knows.

I realise I've been too scared to unleash the real depths of my sadness and anxiety on someone who knows my daughter because I didn't want them to judge. I sometimes feel as though we're not allowed to own our discomfort or pain, or the fact that sometimes being a mum is truly gut-wrenchingly awful because of all the women who would kill to be in our position. We are SO lucky. I realise I am also secure enough in my unequivocal love for my child to sit here now and say, without caveats:

'Sometimes being a mum is really hard.'

Only to Pat, though.

Pat put my foot down and did a kind face at me. *Just tell me what to do,* I inwardly shouted at her. *Tell me how I do all this better, how I can feel strong and good and capable.* There was just silence.

'What if you could say, I want to be ME and I want to be with my daughter? What if you came to a place where you felt like you were fulfilling the *you* bit and the *her* bit at the same time? Maybe that's what you're after: just to find YOU.'

I felt that same feeling I get when I finally find the hook in an article I'm writing, something that shapes a story nicely, giving me a beginning, middle and end to work on.

That doesn't sound selfish, that sort of sounds sensible, actually.

I had a goal: to find out who I was, and that would make me a better parent. But just as quickly as the feeling had flooded my brain, it was gone and I slumped back down. Because that wasn't a goal I could envisage nailing in a couple of sessions of reflexology. I wasn't sure Pat would release my inner powerhouse via my big toe. To find out who I was, to rediscover or even make up a new me could take months, years even. And I kind of need to get it done before nursery starts in four weeks' time since I know deep down that Rich is right – she needs to go.

But imagine falling in love with someone who changes every single week, who moves on and away from you. A friend suggested that you don't feel the wrench initially because you're in complete control – they don't move far without you, they don't fight back against your opinions, they're mostly complicit. It's weird now, because I look back on the first two years and think, that was easy. There was the fog of having a baby weighing me down, but it was a happy fog and people expected so little of me, I expected so little of myself so I didn't question what would come next.

I had been completely broken down by the lack of sleep, the self-doubt, the guilt and the physical changes of the first year and then hastily rebuilt myself in the snatched moments while the baby slept or was with my mum. I couldn't have booked myself a Personal Shopper at Topshop to Gok-Wan me back to myself. There was nothing the reflexologist, my mum or even Rich could have done.

CHAPTER THIRTEEN

I EVENTUALLY SELF-SOOTHE, I THINK

I didn't have a big breakthrough, you know? It wasn't any one thing that brought me back to myself, that helped me piece myself back together. Time just sort of marched on. I think the only conscious change I made was to err on the braver side when making decisions, however small they might seem. Give nursery a go. Return to *Glamour*. Book the holiday. Stay a bit later at the wedding. Get her the scooter …

And gradually, over time, I accepted the constant change with less fear and I tried to plough some of my energy into other things outside of my family. And because everyone else was already on that path and ready for me to catch up, it worked.

My daughter grew up and needed me less urgently. She seemed less vulnerable, somehow. I gained perspective. In time, I did move on. It was slow and never smooth, but it was happening underneath the day-to-day routine and all the mini milestones we were totting up.

'Let's play "I Spy"', I told her, playing for time because the cafe was taking an age to deliver her plate of fish and chips.

'OK, Mama. You do it.'

'OK. I spy with my little eye something beginning with "Fffeeer".'

'Fwog?'

'Nope.'

'Fuck?'

'HEY, NO, NOW –'

'Vodka?'

'WAIT, WHAT?'

Leaving the kid with STRANGERS. On tiny chairs

The first milestone on the horizon was nursery. I had been dreading it, but keeping her away would have been a signal to her and everyone else that I lived in constant fear of her being ill. I knew we should be living life as normal, and this was the first step. So, as this small, dungareed kid turned two and a half, I took her to the nursery we'd signed up for a year before, and as we entered the big playroom, she ran straight into the garden with a swell of what looked like teenagers, they were so big and robust. I saw her little blonde head disappear in amongst the dumper trucks and chalkboards. She didn't look back and the kindly teacher suggested I go and get a coffee and collect her again in an hour. *What, I just hand her over to relative strangers for hours at a time and go … what? Where? And why?* I had no idea how this would work. When my mum was looking after her, I'd be cramming work into every possible second. This woman was suggesting I just have a bit of alone time. What would I do with it?*

From the start, you're warned to bond, you *must* bond! You must have the skin-to-skin, then the co-sleeping and the feeding *and oh God, you must enjoy it all, enjoy!! Treasure each moment!* But now: *OK, separate. Suddenly and without warning you should just leave her somewhere with people you don't really know, and that's good too. Yes, she's crying and you're crying, but it's good, do it, do it!*

Luckily, the kid seemed to like nursery, and she was learning so much so quickly.

The only problem we had was when she went through a phase of punching her classmates – at that stage, all boys – without warning. The teacher reassured us she thought it was pre-emptive as some of the boys were boisterous, but I didn't need the reassurance – I was secretly delighted she could look after herself. We did have the odd occasion when the teacher would peel her off me and I would watch as they carried her out of sight, screaming for me, and I would cry, only to get a phone call before I'd got back to the car to say she was fine.

'Today at nurs'ry, this boy hit me on the head with a truck.'

'NO WAY! What did you do? Did you cry? Did you tell the teacher?'

'No, I hit him on the head with a train.'

'Oh. Um, but we shouldn't ever hit –'

---

* This was when we realised we'd forgotten how many months old she was – when did that happen?! I think we measure time differently in early childhood because the intensity is such that we can't believe it's only been five months and not five years.

'And then he cried and peed his pants and the teacher had to write it down.'

'Uh huh. OK.'

'I think tomorrow I'll play with someone else. I don't want him to pee on me.'

Now, here's the weird thing. The little bite of freedom I got made me crave more. Initially I hated nursery days, but when I realised we could thrive independently, it got quite addictive. Not weird when you consider the fact that for two and a half years I'd barely had more than an hour away from her, even if I was in the next room and my mum was in charge of her wellbeing, I was basically there.

You know when you first start out with a new lover you can't get enough of each other and you dread the day you'll have to spend some time apart? Then you do, and it's amazing because you come back together with anecdotes and new ideas and a fresher armpit, perhaps. I think it was a little bit the same with nursery. I had dreaded it and then when she got in the car full of stories, blushing at the mention of new friends and how much she loved her teacher, I was high as a kite. She was enjoying life and I had mistakenly thought that would only be possible under my watchful eye. So daft – I think I might have narcissistic tendencies … No, really – but there it is.

Sometimes I sat and watched TV; sometimes I'd take a walk. Most of the time I would work, but even that felt luxurious without the limited parameters of nap time and lunches to prepare.

Freedom is the wrong word. I never felt trapped by my child. I never wanted 'out', not once. But it did feel like the possibilities were stretching out in front of me for the first time in a long while.

Working nine to FINE!

I started back at *Glamour*. I enjoyed the hustle and bustle and the importance placed on things that had zip to do with my family. I was contributing to something else, and it felt so good. I needed that familiar setting where I was valued for my work and my opinion to get to grips with this new me.

I developed a small section of wardrobe that contained only 'work clothes' – silk, wool and leather items in pale, stainable colours which were only donned for days in the office, lest The Real World taint them with kid dribble and Dairylea. It was a capsule wardrobe, a mirage of professionalism in amongst the sweats and stained flannel shirts.

I repeatedly turned up to meetings with a very small My Little Pony notebook and a blue crayon to make notes with, because the kid had slipped it in my bag when I was not looking, presumably hiding my grown-up notepad and Bic in the pocket of her bed guard, again.

I missed the after-work drinks and industry parties to rush home to kiss my baby on the head even if she was fast asleep, panic setting in when the train was delayed. I ducked and dived a thousand potential bomb threats at Oxford Circus and spent my lunch break guilt-buying toys and kids' clothes. At work, I was energised and when I returned to my kid to play, I swept through the bath-time routine, keen to fast forward to another exciting day in the office. I was stuck somewhere between feeling quite satisfied and happy, and feeling like I was the worst mum ever.

But I felt stronger every day. And she was having a great time, according to my mum.

'So, she can write her name now, you know.'

'Yes, Mum, we've been working on that together.'

'Hmm. I think I taught her though, really, because we started it months ago. I also taught her to count to 10, you know?'

'Did you? I thought nursery did that the other week?'

'No, all me. And we've been discussing menstruation.'

'Menstruation. Does a three-year-old need to know about that, do you think?'

'Yes, darling. I mean, just the other day I heard her explaining to your dad's friend, Terry, that you were on your period and she saw a bloody tampon in the loo, so I thought it best I explain to her how all that works. Terry chipped in a bit, of course.'

Sure, it smarted a bit when my mum was convinced she was teaching her all the major life skills in one afternoon a week, but it was also kind of a relief, actually: I could share the load.

Weeks into my new job we went out for supper with Lou and her husband and she commented that I seemed like a different person. And I was – I had stories and news to share. I had things to say and the confidence to say them. *Did I just need to get back to work?* I pondered the next day.

She just gets me

Just when I was beginning to piece myself back together, my best mate arrived home from three years in Singapore, with a son who was only four months younger than my daughter. Suddenly, I had a glimpse of a life where the stars do align and you go through it all with a close mate. Once they'd settled into their new home, I was invited over: it would just be us and our babies. We'd Skyped a few times and emailed in the early days before our days got filled to bursting with lactating and purée-ing and nappy changing. I was nervous that she would have changed for the better and would see that I had changed for the worse. That she wouldn't be finding it as hard as I was, that all my insecurities wouldn't match up to hers and we'd realise we no longer had anything in common.

The minute she opened the door, I knew that even if I dropped my kid on her head and wet myself, Natasha would pick us both up, wipe us down and promise not to mention it to Rich. We knew each other before babies and so could be completely honest about how hard it all was without fear of judgement, because we KNEW the core of each other. She saw how I'd changed without judging and understood how it had all happened because it had happened to her too. She unwittingly played such a huge role in bringing me back to myself, because I remembered who I had been, the better bits, and was able to cobble together a reformatted version – like an iPhone update – with her help and support. That was bloody lucky, and such good timing.

'You're such a good mum,' she said one day. I blinked back tears and punched her arm, obviously.

Luckily, Natasha and a new friend, Jo – the older sister of a school friend who had just moved down from London – shared so many of my stunted ambitions and confused feelings of guilt; they both got it. Each woman brought relief that I wasn't alone with my weird feelings and empowered me with each step forward they took. Every guilt-ridden episode felt more like a great anecdote. They helped me to realise that the pressure to EMBRACE EVERY SECOND of time spent with your child is ridiculous and only serves to make time away impossible to enjoy.

They helped me to feel more equipped for my experience of motherhood. When the kids were occupied, Natasha and I would try and work out what it was we wanted from parenthood.

'So, I've ditched the parenting books and have tried reading a bit of the Dalai Lama –'

'What, the guy who's never had kids and basically hangs out with supermodels and world leaders all day long?'

'Yeh, but he's like very *Chicken Soup for the Soul*, isn't he? Anyway, he said, "Caring for others is the best way to fulfil our own interests." And that's how you feel when they're newborn, isn't it? That full-on caring mode is really fulfilling. So why is it that three years in, when caring for her doesn't require such constant action, I want him to add something like, "… if those interests are solely based in care." I know, I know – he's saying they *should* be based solely in care, that it's the only way to feel fully whole. But I also get a lot of satisfaction from self-serving activities and thoughts, OK?' I felt selfish and guilty as soon as I said it.

'Yeh, because we still get fulfilment from gin and work and Netflix.'

'Yes, exactly. OK, good.'

But I kept on trying to untangle this knot, picking away at the tightest bits so I could get a grip on what was going on with me. Caring for others isn't the same as self-sacrifice – you can't take care of someone well unless you take care of yourself. You have to find a way that makes you happy, too. It turned out I couldn't sustain the Earth Mother I was during the first year because it's not how I always want it to be. I can't always hold my crying child to my breast because she wants to scream and kick things for a bit. I can't spend every night rocking my child to sleep because I haven't the patience.

You do whatever it takes to protect, nourish and support this child, and love makes a lot of that easy and instinctive. But there still comes a point when a lot of us will hit a wall. And the true friends that make it out of this jungle alive with you won't judge you for that. Because it's the judgement that really destroys a woman. Whether it's the tuts when you hand your iPad to your kid in a restaurant for five minutes to shore up your relationship with your partner, the eye-roll when you hand over a lollipop to stem a tantrum in your over-tired toddler.

Just because we are parents, it doesn't mean that any of us have the right to judge or criticise.

Raising a feminist

I am constantly refining my own sense of how I can contribute to the feminist agenda. On a daily basis. Because despite grumpy folk telling us we've won the war already and it's time to stop whingeing, I feel more strident than ever. Because I have this new woman to think of. The slights, the injustices and the inequality at stake is driving her future as much as mine. I don't want her to be paid less or discriminated against – I don't want there to be limits imposed. And I don't want her to have to worry like I did.

I listened when my parents told me to dress carefully so as not to attract the wrong kind of attention, i.e. rape. I knew I shouldn't walk anywhere alone at night, that I should text somebody when I got into a cab or the bus alone. It was almost second nature – don't be racist, don't steal stuff, don't lead men on. But when I sat back to think about the implications for my own daughter, it drove me insane. Why are we asking girls to take responsibility for the actions of men? I'm fairly sure it's not rogue women we're worried about when they're crossing the park in a pair of hot pants. How is the bad behaviour of men so ingrained in us that we feel the best way to deal with it is to prepare girls for the inevitability of it? So that when a boy first forced my hand into his pants when I was 16, I assumed I had lead him on. And when the same boy initiated sex in a similarly clumsy way years later, I went along with it, to be polite. I barely moved, and ran away from him as soon as it was over. I felt changed. My first experience of sex was with a kind and gentle long-term boyfriend, who set the bar for it being something wholly positive and mutually desired. But even so, for a short while I began to see sex as something men wanted and took from women; we were to acquiesce. And this was when Sex and the City was all the rage! Nuts.

I don't want my daughter to ever feel that way. So yes, I'm angry and loud. Look, to shift things we *have* to be angry! We have to be loud! It has to be enough to tip the balance that's been the status quo for the longest time. It has to be intersectional and it has to be something you fight for, snarl over and mouth off about every single day. You have to tell your child's teachers, your friends and anyone else who'll listen.

Still married

At some point, through all of this, I realised just how pivotal to my sanity Rich had been, and how rather than acknowledging it, I'd often just sort of taken it for granted. Without any great moment or speech to set us on another path, we just seemed to come back together. Mainly because we've slept a bit more. We have got the negotiations over 'free time' down: he gets curry nights with his mate and I get Sunday mornings to sleep in until 9am. Well, sort of – once he's asked me about 28 questions about what to feed the kid, whether she eats strawberries or not and whether the porridge should be hot or cold. And the two of them mostly watch TV together until I finally get up and have to clean everywhere, thanks to their quickly abandoned Play-Doh slaughterhouse.

Sometimes we are silently negotiating right down to who does the hair wash versus who does the teeth-brushing. Other times we are like the old us and take all of it on so the other can rest, or else parent like Morecambe and Wise preparing break-fast to 'Bring Me Sunshine'. I think my needs are far simpler these days – *tell me I'm doing an OK job and I'll probably blow you*. It's why I spend so long telling him about the games I've played and the play dates I've survived. I don't need a medal exactly, and I'm aware our kid's happiness and enjoyment should be the only reward I need. But sometimes a cup of coffee wouldn't go amiss either.

I regularly feel like I've lost a year somewhere due to sleep deprivation. I honestly get my age wrong every time and when I told Rich that our neighbour has been ribbing me about our impending seven-year itch, he said,

'Bubs, we've been married for eight years.'

'Hmm … Really? OK, sure. I'll just write that down somewhere …'

We seem to agree on most things, other than the utensils drawer in the kitchen, which seems to be the catalyst for most parenting rows. You know the sort – full of wooden spoons and spatulas we never use, with a section for candles from every birthday we've ever had where we go, oh look, we've hardly burnt that down, we'll keep that for next time. There were around 98 candles at last count. Anyway, this drawer has a propensity to pop its base from the frame, and spoons and spatulas go crashing down into the cupboard below. Rich has fixed it several times now, but every so often it slyly slips itself out again and it makes him really cross. As I've mentioned, very little gets Rich cross, so this drawer has become a metaphor for the things about me and our lives that frustrate him. It's a meta-drawer. He blames me for the breakage – I am overfilling the drawer apparently, although it was HIS birthday most recently, so those extra two candles are actually HIS fault, but no matter. We very rarely argued in the old days, and now? We argue over a drawer.

Interestingly, rows about the utensil drawer tended to coincide with a dry patch in conjugal relations, and so I'd been thinking it was time for another stab at sex. 'STAB' BEING THE OPERATIVE WORD.

It was weird to discover how much I had reverted back to almost virginal status after a dry spell. I had to be re-educated.

And I don't mean with diagrams of the penis or practising blowjobs on a beer bottle. I mean, finding out what turns you on and how to get enthusiastic about sex. As a 17-year-old virgin, I was terrified of sex and not at all worried about whether I'd be turned on or not, just that I get it done with as little pain as possible. Well, I felt the same post-baby, but this time I knew there was the potential for it to be great, and I didn't want to just put up with it being painful or a one-sided process. So, just as I'd plugged my earphones into my tiny television in the middle of the night as a teenager to sit, wide-eyed, watching *Sexetera* and *Eurotrash*, once again we were back in front of the TV at random o'clock, seeing if anything in *Game of Thrones* would kick-start my sexuality again.

'Hmm, maybe you could do a Khal Drogo kind of thing?' I suggested one night.

Rich growled. 'DROGO GRRRR!'

'He wouldn't say his own fucking name, you knob!'

'Um … GRRRR, DRAGONS!'

'Oh, just forget it.'

The feelings I experienced when abstaining from sex were all those I swore I'd never give into – guilt that I wasn't giving Rich something he enjoyed and I was solely allowed to give, worries that it would jeopardise our relationship – all the things I internally mocked when friends had felt the same way in the past. Because as a feminist I believed in MUTUAL enjoyment of sex – don't do it for any other reason than desire. And didn't this apply to married sex? In my head maybe more so, since I always shunned the bits of marriage which cast women as the submissive or obeying party. But it turns out those feelings are organic when you love someone. I did feel guilty. I didn't miss the sex all that much if I'm honest – I think the insane love rushes I was experiencing with my kid covered those bases for me, and I just couldn't feel sexual in my own body. Not just the way it looked – so old and so unfamiliar – but because of the way it felt. It was sore and heavy with tiredness. I was incredibly aware of my vagina, so that even when the bruising had vanished and it was basically healed, it was almost as though I had a kind of phantom flap pain.

'Rich, will you get your hand OUT of my pants, I am trying to do the washing-up. WHY do you always grope me when the chances of me being aroused are slim to none?'

'What?! You just looked sexy from the back.'

'Oh, that's really great, that is! So I look better from behind, AND when I'm soaping up a roasting tin which basically renders me defenceless. God, you're such a bloody pervert.'

I am apparently at my sexiest while simultaneously washing up and trying to coax the kid into finishing her pudding. While bent over the toy box, trying to find my phone. Once, when I was unzipping to go to the loo.

So his advances inevitably cast me as the frigid cow and him as the spurned lover who was just trying his best. But, NO! Pick your moments and make me WANT to say 'yes', you know? Really, he was just trying to work an opportunity but I was not amused.

He changed tack, buying me a bra and knickers from Agent Provocateur, knowing my stance on cheap pants ('These are manufactured by the same people who sell thrush remedies, Rich, I guarantee it,' I'd explain, repurposing said pants into dusters). This was a beautiful dark blue set, though – sheer but for the scarlet flowers embroidered across the cup. I squealed as I unwrapped the pink box, and held the bra aloft, its intricate design so beautiful and delicate in comparison to my thick cotton nursing bras. I removed more black tissue paper and found the knickers – cute little bikini briefs … with absolutely no gusset.

'Dude, are these … crotchless?' I stuck two fingers through the hollow where the crotch should have been.

Rich looked confused. 'Um, no … I wouldn't buy crotchless, bubs. I know you wouldn't want that.'

He brought up the website on his phone and scanned down to the dark blue panties.

'See!' I pointed below the picture, 'Ouvert! That means "open".'

'Oh,' he looked crestfallen, 'I thought that was the name of the colour.'

I did wear them once, but with my abbreviated labia, only one side peeked through the 'ouvert' bit. There was something very comforting, though, about that pink box sitting on top of our wardrobe, a reminder that I could still own pretty, impractical things that were sexy but not in a battery-powered way. And that Rich still thought I'd look good in scanties, I suppose.

It was as if there was a switch in my brain that needed to be flicked back on. All the intention would be there in the morning, and would continue through the day – *I want to show this man how much I love him, I know it'll be good, I know it'll be worth it* – then I'd get into bed and quite often freeze. My mum-brain still insisted on an early night, and no fanny business. *You're tired,* it says, *sleep is more important.* I wanted it to take less effort, for it to be less of a chore. I wanted to melt into him, for it not to be so carefully stage-managed and kind of brutal.

Thankfully, in time my vagina was suitably stretched. Sex eventually grew easier and nicer. Some very irresponsible bare-back sex proved to be the breakthrough – literally – and once I stopped breastfeeding, sex was almost back to normal. As promised, it did bring a semblance of natural desire back, so that's good. It was a physical transaction as much as an emotional one – as the intensity of my child's reliance on me ebbed away, I had space for another person. And I realised I *needed* to be sexual because when you're a mum it's something that's just for *you* (and your partner, if you're feeling generous). Especially for someone like me who doesn't get a buzz from exercise or hobbies. Your body languishes untouched. Sex helps connect you back to the person you were before, to connect to your partner. I learnt that we thrive when we're physically close. We can abstain, but only if we agree why and when and for how long so there's no resentment or rejection. For us, that held for about three months then we were forever on different planes, trying to match the other desire for desire, but often just power-ing through for the sake of the other.

Eventually I started to feel a bit less 'my vagina is mashed', a bit more, 'my vagina has changed – deal with it'. I think possibly because I was reading a lot of Lena Dunham stuff and I knew that if she saw it, she would just like shrug, as in, 'Big whoop, mine's been on TV'. As time went on and I realised it was less likely to prolapse, I felt less mumsy, more like my old self. It's the interim years before it gets really saggy or wrinkly, I assume, and I should just enjoy it more now, before it's a dry husk of its former self.

So, four years later, I suppose my sexual self is back but so different. We're always way more grateful when we do get laid – like anything that's eked out having been scoffed to the max, you savour each moment and dine out on the memory of those morsels for hours.

Shall we have another?

Oh, hell no.

'When are you going to have another? And another and another and another?' SUCH a fucking inappropriate question. I mean, what if we're trying to get pregnant and it's just not happening? What if I'm midway through the eighth miscarriage since our daughter was born? What if it's just impossible? What if we are just not having sex anymore and are on the verge of a break up? What if we can't afford it? I don't think there is a worse question, and one pertaining to your gynaecological, sexual and financial wellbeing that's thrown around with such gay abandon by every Tom, Dick and Twat going.

This isn't a new question – it was asked as soon as our daughter was born, presumably to gauge how you felt about the newborn phase, and it's tricky to say with conviction, NEVER! Because either the person will tell you you'll change your mind (oh, OK), or you sound like your current baby is such a nightmare, it's put you off for life. So there's no point in me answering that question honestly, and instead I tend to say something elusive like, 'Never say never!'

The truth is, we'd always said we'd just have one child, when we talked about the hypothetical children we'd expect in our late thirties. I'm basically an only child (my six half-siblings from my dad's first marriage were raised quite separately), I liked it that way and once I pointed out the financial benefits of sticking to one, Rich was quite keen too. In fact his only concern – as one of three kids – was that she'd be lonely sometimes. But I was never lonely: I was with my parents or with friends, and equally happy playing alone.

But when our daughter was born, I wavered. *This perfect creature, this amazing rush, this incredible experience – why would I pass up the opportunity to do this a second, or even a third time?! Why would I make this a one-time thing when it made me and everyone around me SO happy?* Rich was unmoved, arguing that our daughter was what had made it such a happy experience – if we couldn't count on replicating her exactly, it couldn't be as good a second time around.

I wrote an article about it for *The Guardian* and just happily chirruped my reasons for only having one child as per the editor's suggestion. I didn't think about how my agenda might differ to others' or that the editor would want a strident argument rather than someone umming and ahhing, so when I saw the final edit of the story through the eyes of over 300 angry commenters, I realised I should keep my mouth shut. Especially as the truth is I have no idea if I want another one or not! But that does not make for good copy, of course.

Rich and I still talk about it a lot. I often throw out a 'AWW, I wanna have another baby!' when there's one on TV or I see a baby picture of our daughter. We find it hard to see her grow up and out of the baby phase because it feels too soon. To grow out of phases and leave them behind forever, knowing we won't relive it all with a second baby. I ask her if she wants a brother or sister and she turns up her nose at the very suggestion, which is a huge relief, even if she is only four and basically shouldn't be tasked with this kind of decision.

Ultimately, if we had a repeat of 1 January 2012, I'd be down with it. I'd do all the hypnobirthing. I'd take photos of my bump. I'd embrace it, knowing what comes of such a process. I keep telling myself things like, *You've still got years to decide* and *Maybe if we ever have a bit more money*. Other days I think, *No, it wouldn't benefit any of us*. Then I think, OHMYGOD WHERE WILL SHE GO FOR CHRISTMAS IF RICH AND I BOTH DIE?

The thing is, I'd be doubly scared if we did go ahead and try for another baby. I had such an innate sense of peace when I was pregnant, I knew it would all turn out OK. I wasn't scared of labour, I wasn't scared for her or for me, I knew it would be OK. But also, I knew NOTHING about pregnancy or birth. Next time I would be scared. I would worry about that kid, about all the things that could go wrong now I know more, I know better. I would also worry about my first born. I know I could love another, for sure. But how would she feel? If I imposed a complete cataclysmic change on her life as she knew it.

'I'm not going to get married, Mama, because I always want to live with you.'

'Ah, that's nice, baby, but you might want to have your own baby one day.'

'No, I won't because they come out of your vagina and it hurts.'

'Oh. Well, but you might want to live with your friends. I did that and it was really fun.'

'Nah. When you're old I want to hold your hand and drive you to Sainsbury's and plait your hair for you.'

How could I not want eight of these people in my life, when I have the option?

But also, I now know how much it costs, financially and emotionally. And I love that I came back to myself, to a new career and a fresh try at being me. You know, without having to go to prison first or rehab or a yoga retreat. My daughter has brought me to myself, she points out on a daily basis the best version of me, when I don't rush and hurry, where I take joy in silliness and her sweet face. I get it all from her.

It's tough to admit but I like how things have fallen now in peace. I do worry about her being lonely, but I also see the benefits of her getting us to herself, I guess. We couldn't have a baby based solely on the fact that it *might* make her happier, because we know so many sibling relationships which haven't worked out that well, so we see it as a huge risk that we'd need to make major compromises to even attempt. She has a lot of cousins, so … Yep, that's what we keep telling ourselves.

And so we recoil from the fun suggestion we do it all again. I regret it when I see siblings being sweet to one another and try to remember how much I liked being an only child. Every time a friend announces she's pregnant, I feel something weird. There's the joy but tinged with a smidgen of jealousy, I think.

I also think I have a false sense of how long we have to change our minds. I'm 34 this year, so I give myself another 10 years. That somehow provides some comfort. But still – we're not having another, OK? Nope, definitely not. Mm mm. Well, OK, MAYBE, but probably not. Oh God.

ME

I had always been very into pigeon-holing myself – I think most people who grew up with the Spice Girls are – it was the simplest way to identify myself. Stay-At-Home Mum. Attachment Parent. Scary Mum, Sporty Mum. Cool Mum. Still-Got-It Mum. Private Mum. Public Mum. But quite often it was also the cause of the fight inside my brain because actually there was no one-size-fits-all label I could sit under and they all seemed to be at odds with one another. I wanted to be relaxed but I was naturally neurotic. I wanted to be the party girl but I was knackered. I wanted to be intellectually stimulated and still contribute to the world beyond our living room, but I was knackered.

So, I'm slummy with a side of precious, I'm uptight and naughty; I'm a composite of the mums I've met and loved, as well as the bits I thought I'd never be.

I am pretty consistent. In that I consistently type 'toddler slushy poo slightly green' into Google in the hope that it'll throw up something comforting when I am staring down a potential 24 hours of explosive gastric disease. I am looking forward to a new milestone if it promises more sleep and less paraphernalia and then mourning the passing of a phase because it spelled out the brevity of childhood and this sweet, uncomplicated relationship with a baby.

I'm prat-falling in the supermarket, rolling down grassy inclines when it's been raining, making inappropriate noises in the doctor's waiting room, because nowadays that's what counts. I cover for her when she cops a squat behind the bar at our friend's wedding because she just can't hold it any longer. I'm leaving the house wearing three Peppa Pig hair clips and two stickers on my cheek, but I'm not a twat, I'm a hero. I'm *her* hero. When we go to New York as a family for the first time I realise how cool The American Museum of Natural History is. She wanders over to the sculpture of Theodore Roosevelt sitting on the bench and holds his hand, gazing up at his serious face with reverence. I see how the trees in Central Park are perfect for napping under, and how the dancers on The Highline are worth all the dollar bills our daughter pulls from our pockets for them. It breaks my heart when she says,

'Grandpa would love it here, wouldn't he, Mama?'

As a woman, I am finding time to consider what else I am. I have a space in my life where I'm not a mum, where I am redis-covering my sexuality, where I love working and am trying to be a better friend. I have clear-cut opinions sometimes, and I have goals beyond a smooth bedtime. I'm less of a people pleaser. Well, now it's for the greater good, AKA my kid, I cancel, I ghost and I make it awkward. And although it sounds horrible, I'm actually really proud of that development in my character: it's like a social backbone I didn't have before.

And I live in hope.

Hope that one day interrupted sleep will be a distant memory that we only remember because we're so well rested and our brains work perfectly again.

That the final 75 per cent push of the sale season will feature my daughter's shoe size.

That we'll have more sex.

That my mum and mother-in-law know how much I appre-ciate their love, despite my sometimes gruff nature.

That I'll be more patient tomorrow.

That my kid never becomes seriously ill.

That she'll be a happy school child, a happy teenager and have a wonderful life.

Nothing major's happened, really, to make me feel fully formed again. Or at least, the things that *have* happened have been noteworthy for reasons outside of motherhood. The weddings we've been to, the work trips I've taken, the honest and frank conversations I finally had the guts to initiate with Rich, my parents and my friends. But really, it's been about time. Time passing, first at a starling rate, then more gradually, teaching me by rote with every curveball thrown at me that everything's a phase and change is just round the corner. You don't have to have it all figured out. It's all been key to coming back to myself, a new, more accepting self.

I can't do an EAT-PRAY-LOVE style getaway to find myself. I want to find it all here, with these two people I love. Sometimes you have to lose yourself to find yourself, and gradually I'm finding myself right here. Rather than feeling like I'm past my prime and unseen by the outside world, I feel seen more intently than ever by my child.

Now, school looms on the horizon, our toddler becomes a child and I'm less scared of what that means for us three, I'm excited. I'm gutted – our baby is going to be somewhere else Monday–Friday from now on – but I'm also excited.

I had to figure out how to raise her AND myself. I'm getting there.

THE AFTERBIRTH

Next week I'll turn 34. Rich always gets a bit twitchy at this time of year because I expect a LOT on my birthday these days and he rarely knows what these expectations involve until AFTER the fact, when I will sulk and point out what he *could* have done differently. Although we're sitting side by side on the sofa we're basically in our own little worlds as I'm writing on my laptop and Rich is doing a bad job of disguising the fact he's trying to Amazon Prime me a birthday present and failing miserably. Finally, he pipes up:

'What do you want to do for your birthday?'
    'I don't mind, bubs.'
    'We could go away for the weekend?'
    'Hmm, maybe.'
    'We could go to Florence? Or just keep it local, maybe London?'
    'That sounds nice.'
    'And we could even try that thing we've been talking about? Maybe it's time for that?!'

'My mum says it really hurts and isn't really worth the mess.'

'Well, then let's try it and see if she's right?'

'Fuck off, Rich.'

This is an interesting conversation because it could have taken place before we had a baby, but until recently it would never have fitted into our new lives as parents. There's no mention of our kid in this conversation, and Rich's suggestion that we go away is genuine and realistic. By the power of babysitters and an independent four-year-old who loves sleepovers at her granny's house, all the rest of the birthday proposal is technically possible. When I was about to turn 30, the question 'what do you want to do for your birthday?' was all it took for me to unravel. But now? It's all possible. Apart from THAT THING, obviously. Not happening. I'm not even sure how you get a leg to bend that way.

I'm a million miles from who I used to be. For a long time I felt ashamed of every negative feeling, or that I felt harmed by the experience. It's crazy how it works. It's the most intense, pure and beautiful love that simultaneously makes you feel better than you could have imagined feeling and wracked with the pulsing fear that it's your responsibility to keep this perfect person alive and well in an increasingly hostile world.

As our children grow, the routine can simply push you further under, as the cycle of care and sustenance spins away – whether or not it is punctuated by work. You lose those quiet, solitary moments, as well as the moments where your sense of self is mirrored by those around you. Instead you are constantly surrounded by noise or worry, and yet with these constant companions you feel alone. Like nobody hears you. And you can't really complain, because this has been the job of parents since time immemorial, and what did you expect? You're supposed to give your whole self over to it. Your story seems to be ending with this greater good in mind, with someone more worthy of effort and care.

It's taken me ages to write those words and leave them there. I want my daughter to know how much I enjoyed the first four years, how she changed my life for the better. That it was just *me* who couldn't keep up with this rush of change. The negative aspects of the experience – frustration, self-doubt, fear – they were all *my* weaknesses. I want her to know about the umpteen times she made me laugh and cry with pure love, how miraculous she is, how many astounding moments I've had since she was born that blow every single momentous moment before her birth out of the water. How nothing has made me happier than being her mother and that it's the most important thing in my life. Yes, it's true. I could lose it all – career, home, entire family – and it would suck but as long as I had her, I'd be fine. Without her there would be no me, because there's no way I could continue to exist.

But what I am saying here – and I hope will one day be helpful to her too, should she decide to have kids – is that there might be a way to make yourself as important in your life as your child, to regain balance and that in doing so, you become a better mum. Frustratingly, you can't seek it out or work for it. You have to just be in your new life and allow it to come to you.

I know – it's definitely easier said than done. But believe me, it's also easier than constantly floundering under the strongest of currents, trying to do it all and be the best at everything. I'm trying, and it's better.

Could I have done this when she was a newborn and dependent on me for everything? Honestly? No. Could I have made this change sooner? Absolutely. I am irretrievably changed and I am no longer in control – her journey is affecting me all the time. It's steering me. The mother-of-a-newborn and the mother-of-a-toddler me were different, and the next 'me' will be too. But I will have the independence and assurance to know that the next hurdle will pass just like the last.

This identity crisis takes hold when you're subsumed by the everyday challenges and minutiae of parenting, no matter how seemingly unthreatening those challenges might be. And it hits you when you're down, dragged under to a greater level of vulnerability by lack of sleep and confidence, without the armour of friends, colleagues or familiarity. You may start arguing with the one you love, suddenly feel criticised by them or find them unexpectedly lacking. You might feel a wedge being driven between you or look over the Moses basket at them and wonder, who even are you? Or if you're alone, you might lose sight of where your baby's needs end and you start.

And no matter how well read you are, no matter how hard you've studied, every child is an unknown quantity and can completely defeat the most in control of parents with a single red cheek or late bowel movement. Everyone experiences that moment when you've run out of ideas and despair that you're letting your baby down. That you're just a bit shit. The thing is, we're a generation of smart, goal-orientated women, who know how to set targets – be they social, professional or physical – and how to work through them systematically. But how do you know you're making a success of motherhood? It's so hard to define successful parenting, and with every little setback it's easy to feel like a failure or that you're incomplete.

Whether you're a stay-at-home mum juggling your child's infinite needs with an active inner life and are no longer defined by the workplace and your working relationships, or a working mum spinning all the plates that keep your family afloat, we can all relate to the changes that can unsteady us as women.

I still haven't worked out what it is I ultimately want. The thing is, to go back to that pre-baby life wouldn't fulfil me. It did at the time – I'm not belittling that life – but it wouldn't allow for the beautiful thing I've got going on with my daughter, with our unit of three, and I prefer that life now. And this restless craving for something else? It feels that everything is within reach now, that life is for the taking again, that I've gained back a little control.

I can sense that the next curveball is on its way. It wasn't the start of school, or the fifth birthday, though. No, the real curveball will be something totally unexpected. Because at the moment I am that wise, all-knowing mum who has done the baby and toddler years and can calmly pass on all my wisdom with a peaceful smile on my lips. And the woman next door with the 13-year-old daughter is chuckling to herself, thinking, 'Oh, you just wait, Timothy! You just wait …'

ACKNOWLEDGEMENTS

My agent Nelle Andrew helped me shape the entire premise of this book. Thank you, Nelle, you took me by the hand and put me on the path I'd been trying to find for years. There's nobody I'd rather have in my corner. I'm looking forward to teaching your baby all the swear words.

Vicky, Julie and Polly. Obviously I'm into you because you're amazing at what you do, but the fact we're a team of new-ish mums is ridiculously on-brand. Thanks for being endlessly enthusiastic and kind. Mums lifting mums. Thank you, Holly and Ellie – that was a weird but great day! Thank you HarperCollins, it's such a huge honour to make a book with you.

Rich. You got me all kinds of knocked up. Nobody's ever got me that knocked up before. Thanks for supporting me, being patient throughout and for showing our daughter the best example of how a man should treat a woman. We are both bloody lucky to have you. I love you.

Mum, Dad: I wouldn't have done very much of anything if it wasn't for you. But on top of the childcare, you have always made me think I'm funnier, prettier, smarter and taller than I actually am. None of life's knocks have done the damage they surely should have done thanks to you making me feel solid and worthwhile. I love you.

Thank you, Doza (and entire Holmes-Hobbs family) for the love, for putting up with me and never actually telling me I'm bonkers. I hope this is the only bit of the book you're going to read, though.

THANK YOU TO THE WOMEN: Poppy Mardall and Natasha Bailie, you are two of the best humans I ever met. Thank you to Nikki, Jo, Hattie, Iso, Marianne, Donna, Clemmie, Lou, Mars, Sharon, Jossel, Barbie, Mia, Dominique and Becky. For the genuinely amazing advice: Stephanie Modell, Mary Atkinson, Bianca Presto, Mary-Kate Trevaskis, Caroline Hirons and Sarah Turner. Helen Whitaker for going above and beyond with the edits, smart insights and virtual hand-holding. To Alessandra: thank you for giving me chance after chance after chance. AND THE MEN: Martin, Steve, Ian, Chris, Jenks, Chuck, Alex and Ollie Blackaby. Thank YOU. And thanks for making me feel less devo about having to be on the book cover: Emily and Izzy at Imagination PR; Jo and Olivia at TCS; Mark at John Frieda, Sarah-Jane Wai for Charlotte Tilbury Beauty and Jo Tutchener-Sharp at Scamp & Dude.